Fundamentals of
GCP and Clinical Research

Fundamentals of
GCP and Clinical Research

Sanjay Gupta

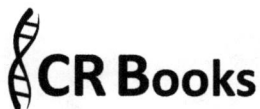

First published in India by
CR Books Pvt. Ltd.
503, NDM-2, Netaji Subhash Place, Pitampura, New Delhi 110034
Tel: +91-11-45121445 Fax: +91-11-45121435
E-mail: info@crbooks.net, info@crbooks.us
Web: www.crbooks.net

First Edition: August 2013
Copyright© CR Books Pvt. Ltd.

The author and publisher have made a conscientious effort to ensure that
the information contained in this book is accurate and in accordance
with the accepted standards at the time of publication. However,
in this rapidly changing world guidelines and practices are
subject to change without prior notification, therefore
readers are advised to confirm these as and
when needed.

ISBN -978-81-9222-77-2-6

Contents

Appendices

Appendix-1. List and Location of Essential Trial Documents
Before the Clinical Phase of the Trial Commences

Appendix-2. List and Location of Essential Trial Documents
During the Clinical Conduct of a Trial

Appendix-3. List and Location of Essential Trial Documents
After Completion or Termination of the Trial

List of Contributors

1. Dr. Surendra H Bodakhe
2. Dr. Munish Ahuja
3. Dr. Vijay Juyal

Preface

Diseases are the major cause of death, disability and sufferings worldwide. Emergence of new diseases having no effective prevention or control as well as growing resistance to available drugs poses a serious threat to mankind.

Clinical trials are the mainstay for bringing out newer, better and safe medicines to serve the mankind. It is the most expensive and time consuming component of the drug discovery process and constitute approximately 70% of the total time and money spent in the overall development process. Typically it takes approximately 12 years and millions of dollars to bring one new drug from conception to market out of which 6-7 years are spent in various phases of clinical trials. The first documented evidence of clinical trial dates back to 1747 when James Lind discovered citrus fruit as a cure for scurvy. The present day clinical trials are conducted in four different phases (I, II, III, and IV). Each phase of clinical trial is aimed at addressing a scientific question with phase-I establishing the initial safety and later phases establishing the efficacy along with the safety. Since, clinical research requires a specific skills set for carrying out various activities, a need of training exists at the level of individual stakeholder.

This book is intended to provide a fundamental knowledge on clinical research and Good Clinical Practice (GCP) guidelines. I hope the book will leave the desired impression and readers would be able to incorporate the learning into practice.

15th August 2013   Sanjay Gupta

1

Introduction to Clinical Research

According to ICH-GCP Guidelines, Clinical Research refers to an investigation on human subjects intended to discover or verify the clinical, pharmacological and/or other pharmacodynamic effects of an investigational product(s), and/or to identify any adverse reactions to an investigational product(s), and/or to study absorption, distribution, metabolism, and excretion of an investigational product(s) with the object of ascertaining its safety and /or efficacy.

In today's scientific era research is taking a major stride in all streams and newer and better drugs are being introduced to cure ailments, which are difficult to treat. Clinical trials are the mainstay for bringing out new drugs to the market and constitute approximately 70% of the total time and money spent in drug development. Typically it takes approximately 12 years and US$ 1 billion to bring one new drug from conception to market out of which 6 to 7 years are usually spent in various phases of clinical trials. In order to develop a comprehensive understanding on clinical research, it is important to understand the overall drug discovery process.

Drug Discovery Process

The drug discovery process begins with the generation of a new idea that is targeted towards chemically modifying a disease process via a drug. The idea is usually generated from a comprehensive understanding of a disease process and a continuing involvement with research in specific therapeutic area of interest. The first step is selection and validation of a 'Target' which is followed by selection of 'Drug' that has the ability to interact with the target.

- **Target selection** involves choosing a disease to treat and then developing a model for that disease. Thus researcher first select or discover a biological target that the scientific team believes may be linked to a pathologic process. It is estimated that up to 10 genes contribute to multi-factorial diseases. These disease genes are further linked to another 5 to 10 gene product in physiological and pathophysiological pathways leading to an availability of approximately 10,000 potential drug targets.

- **Target validation** involves demonstration of relevance of the target protein in a disease process.

- **Drug selection** or Lead selection is a process that involves finding a drug or group of drugs which has the ability to interact with target protein and modulate its activity. Tens of thousands of potential drug substances (obtained from massive compound libraries) are tested against the target proteins in a robotic process called High Throughput Screening (HTS).

- HTS yields Hit compounds that are further studied in detail for their physical,chemical and biological properties. **Hit compounds** with suitable physical,chemical and biological properties are called **Lead candidates.**

- Lead candidates are then chemically modified and pharmacologically characterized to obtain compounds with suitable pharmacodynamic and pharmacokinetic properties to become a drug in a process called **Lead optimization.**

The compound with best profile is then chosen for further investigation in the form of preclinical and clinical testing.

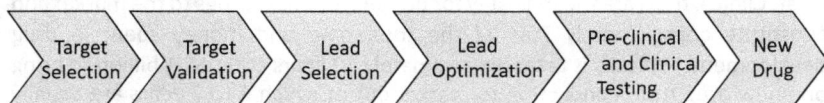

Target Selection	Target Validation	Lead Selection	Lead Optimization	Pre-clinical and Clinical Testing	New Drug

Figure 1 : Drug Discovery Process

Preclinical Testing

Preclinical tests are performed in the laboratory, using a wide array of chemical and biochemical assays, cell-culture models and animal models. The pharmacological activity of every new compound is carefully evaluated. As experience of the compound increases, experimental steps and methods may be modified. Eventually a compound is selected for development. At the pre-clinical stage, the regulatory bodies will generally ask, at a minimum that research team/company must:

(i)   develop a pharmacological profile of the drug.

(ii) determine the acute toxicity of the drug in at least two species of animals.

(iii) conduct short-term toxicity studies ranging from 2 weeks to 3 months, depending on the proposed duration of use of the substance in the clinical studies.

Thus Preclinical Testing Involves:

- Pharmacology testing
- Toxicology testing
- Animal pharmacokinetics testing

Clinical Development of Drug

The Clinical Development Plan

The clinical development plan contains a summary of the pre-clinical findings and of market research done for the drug. It consists of summaries or outlines of studies that will be conducted, target dates for the studies, the objective of each study and the proposed study design for achieving the objective. It also covers the studies required for the registration and approval of the drug.

Phases of Clinical Research

Clinical testing of a drug is done in four phases (I, II, III and IV) of clinical trials. The knowledge gained from one phase is assessed before progressing to the next phase. However, research in a particular phase may continue after the drug has progressed to further stages of development.

- **Phase-I** clinical trials are conducted to establish initial safety, maximum tolerance and pharmacokinetics of a new drug in 20-80 healthy human volunteers (with the exception of cancer drugs where Phase-I trials are done on cancer patients). These are also called as 'First in Man' and acts as a basis of validating the findings from pre-clinical testing in to human beings. Usually Phase-I trials are initiated with a very low dose ($1/10^{th}$ of the optimal animal dose) which is gradually increased to determine the maximum tolerated dose. During Phase-I trials, sufficient information about the drug's pharmacokinetics and pharmacological effects is obtained to plan a well-controlled, Phase-II trial. An Investigational New Drug (IND) Application is filed to regulatory authorities for seeking the permission to initiate Phase-I clinical trials.

- **Phase-II** clinical trials are universally accepted as a standard requirement for the evaluation of efficacy and safety of a new drug. Careful observations are made to determine the dose and adverse reactions in 100-200 patients with the relevant indication. If a new drug is found to be effective and safe in Phase-II trials, it is moved to next phase of development. In case of lack of efficacy the development of drug is stopped at this phase itself.

- **Phase-III** clinical trials are the final pre-marketing phase of clinical trials. These are large, multi-centric trials to establish the safety and efficacy of a new drug vis-à-vis existing standard of care/placebo to form the basis for regulatory submission. If a new drug is found to be safe and effective in Phase-III trials, a New Drug Application (NDA) is filed to regulatory authorities for seeking marketing permission.

- **Phase-IV** clinical trials are post marketing studies that are conducted for generating additional safety data on a drug once it is marketed. Regulatory authorities can withdraw the marketing authorization of a drug anytime if there are safety concerns on its usage.

It is estimated that for every 10,000-30,000 drug molecules screened; only 250-300 enters the pre-clinical testing, 5 enters the clinical testing and 1 reaches to the market.

Phase-I	To establish initial safety and maximum tolerance, pharmacokinetics *etc.* in 20-80 healthy human volunteers. Also called as 'First in Man'.
Phase-II	Universally accepted as a standard requirement for the evaluation of efficacy and safety of the drug. Careful observations are made to determine the dose and adverse reactions in 100-200 patients with the relevant indication *e.g.* randomized, placebo control, blinded *etc.*
Phase-III	Final pre-marketing phase; multi-centric, several patients; safety and efficacy data to establish a drug's risk-benefit relationship; the basis of regulatory submissions.
Phase-IV	Additional safety data; tests the approved drug for additional conditions; expand to much larger patient population.

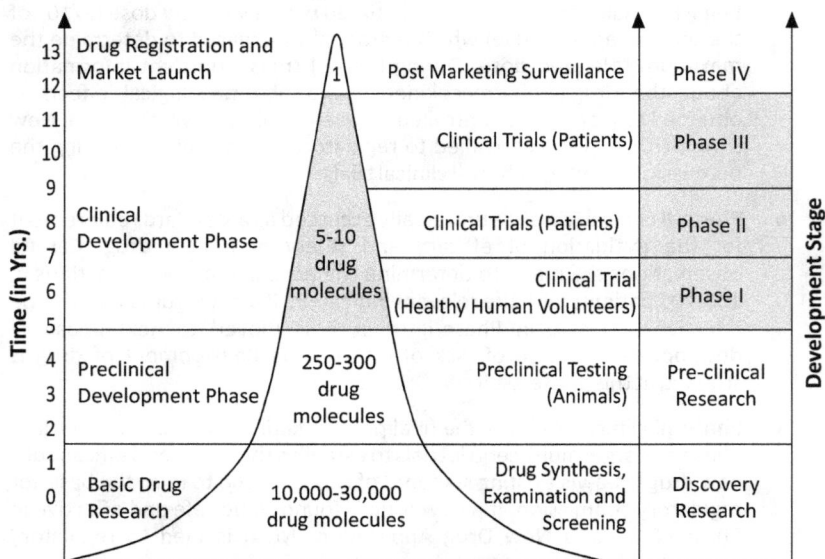

Figure 2: Drug Development Process

2

Evolution of Ethical Research Principles, Regulations and Guidelines

The present day ethical research principles, regulations and guidelines have evolved over a period of time and after a series of scientific misconduct/fraud. Prior to World War II there was very little concern for the participation of human subjects in medical research and therefore there was no formal protection. It started with Nuremberg Code in 1947, the same year when the World Medical Association (WMA) was established.

Nuremberg Code

In 1947 the Nuremberg Code laid down 10 principles to guide physician investigators for experiments involving human subjects. The need to define the basic principles for the conduct of human research was focused towards patient protection and made no distinctions between research with patients and healthy persons, be they prisoners or volunteers. The Nuremberg Code was the result of judgment by an American military war crimes tribunal conducting proceedings against 23 Nazi physicians and administrators for their wilful participation in war crimes and crimes against humanity. The doctors had conducted medical experiments on concentration camp prisoners who died or were permanently affected as a result. The Nuremberg Code was developed in response to the judicial condemnation of the acts of Nazi physicians, and did not specifically address human subject research in the context of the patient-physician relationship.

The 10 principles of the Nuremberg Code are as follows:

1. The voluntary free consent to participate;
2. The experiment to yield fruitful results for the good of society, unprocurable by other methods or means of study;
3. The experiment should be designed based on the results of animal experimentation or other previous work;
4. The experiment should avoid all unnecessary physical and mental suffering and injury;
5. No experiment should be conducted where there is a prior reason to believe that death or disabling injury will occur;

6. The degree of risk to be taken should never exceed that determined by experiment;

7. Proper preparations should be made to protect the experimental subject against even remote possibilities of injury, disability, or death;

8. The research study should be conducted only by scientifically qualified persons;

9. Participants can withdraw from the study at any time;

10. Cessation of study if adverse effects emerges.

Post-Nuremberg Code

Even after Nuremberg Code, the abuse and exploitation of humans in research continued and examples of some of the studies in this regard include:

- Tuskeegee Syphillis Study, 1932-1972
- Thalidomide Disaster, 1962
- Willowbrook School Study, 1963-1966
- Jewish Chronic Disease Hospital Study, 1963

Tuskegee Syphilis Study (1932 1972)

The U.S. Public Health Service (USPHS) conducted a research project from 1932 to 1972 to document the natural progression of syphilis. The subjects of the investigation were poor black sharecroppers from Macon Country, Alabama, with latent syphilis and men without the disease who served as controls. Six hundred low-income African-American males, 399 with latent syphilis and 201 men without the disease were enrolled in the study based on the results of a 1930 venereal diseases control projects survey. This survey had identified Macon Country to have the highest prevalence of Syphilis. The investigators exploited the rural setting of Tuskegee, deprived socioeconomic status, high rates of illiteracy and paucity of medical care during the conduct of study. The physicians conducting the study deceived the participants, telling them that they were being treated for "bad blood" a euphemism for Syphilis. In fact, they deliberately denied treatment to the participants with syphilis and went to extreme lengths to ensure that they would not receive therapy from any other sources. In exchange for their participation, the participants received free meals, medical examination and burial insurance. The rationale for depriving these subjects from receiving curative treatment was that such individuals offer an unusual opportunity to study the untreated Syphilis from the beginning of the disease to the death of the infected person.

The study that lasted for 40 years included only sporadic clinical re-examinations.

By the time the study was exposed in 1972, and ended on November 16th of the same year, 28 men died of syphilis, 100 others were dead due to syphilis related complications, at least 40 women had been infected and 19 children had contracted the disease at birth. On May 16, 1997, U.S. President Bill Clinton apologized, on behalf of the government, to the surviving participants of the Tuskegee Syphilis Study and the members of the Tuskegee Syphilis Study Legacy Committee.

Thalidomide Disaster (1961)

Thalidomide was first introduced in Germany in 1958 as an anticonvulsive agent but soon found unsuitable for this indication. The drug was thought to be useful for a variety of other ailments, including morning sickness caused by pregnancy, hypertension and migraines. By 1961, thalidomide was widely prescribed in Europe. Pregnant women in 48 countries took thalidomide, resulting in the live births of more than 8000 infants affected with severe limb defects and other organ defects. Later, two scientists in Germany (Lenz W. Klinische) and Australia (McBride WG) independently suggested that prenatal exposure to thalidomide was the cause of serious birth defects. Children born to such mothers often were born without arms or with other severe deformities. Thalidomide was sold in a number of countries across the world from 1957 until 1961, when it was withdrawn from the market after being found to be a cause of birth defects in what has been called "one of the biggest medical tragedies of modern times".

Willowbrook School Study (1963 - 1966)

Willowbrook State School, situated in New York State, was an institution for the mentally handicapped children. Parents of children in the institution gave consent for their children to participate in a study. The intent of the research study was to follow the course of viral hepatitis and study the effectiveness of an agent for inoculating against hepatitis. Parents were provided with study information describing the drug administration as vaccinations. However, the children were deliberately infected with the hepatitis virus. Evidence revealed that school admitted only those children to the school whose parents gave permission for them to be in the study.

Jewish Chronic Disease Hospital (1963)

Studies were conducted at the Jewish Chronic Disease Hospital in New York City to develop information on the nature of the human transplant rejection process. Chronically ill patients who did not have cancer were injected with live human cancer cells. The physicians did not inform the patients as to what they were doing. The physician's rationalization for their actions was that "they did not want to scare the patients" and that "they thought the cells would be rejected".

The above abuses and exploitations of humans in research has lead to evolution of more stringent norms such as Declaration of Helsinki, The Belmont Report and ICH-Good Clinical Practice Guidelines.

Declaration of Helsinki

The World Medial Association (WMA) has developed the Declaration of Helsinki as a statement of ethical principles to provide guidance to physicians and other participants in medical research involving human subjects.

Declaration of Helsinki was adopted by the 18th WMA General Assembly, Helsinki, Finland, June 1964 and amended by the 29th WMA General Assembly, Tokyo, Japan, October 1975; 35th WMA General Assembly, Venice, Italy, October 1983; 41st WMA General Assembly, Hong Kong, September 1989; 48th WMA General Assembly, Somerset West, Republic of South Africa, October 1996; 52nd WMA General Assembly, Edinburgh, Scotland, October 2000 and 59th WMA General Assembly, Seoul, October 2008.

The Declaration of Geneva of the WMA binds the physician with the words, "The health of my patient will be my first consideration", and the International Code of Medical Ethics declares that, "A physician shall act only in the patient's interest when providing medical care which might have the effect of weakening the physical and mental condition of the patient". Declaration of Helsinki laid down the Ethical Principles for Medical Research Involving Human Subject and is a major landmark in the evolution of Good Clinical Practices (GCPs).

The basic principles of the Declaration of Helsinki include the following:

- Physician's duty in research is to protect the life, health, privacy, and dignity of the human participant;
- Research involving humans must conform to generally accepted scientific principles and thorough knowledge of scientific literature and methods;
- Research protocols should be reviewed by an independent committee;
- Research protocols should be conducted by medically/scientifically qualified individuals;
- Risks and burden to the participant should not outweigh benefits;
- Researcher should stop study if risks are found to outweigh potential benefits;
- Research is justified only if there is a reasonable likelihood that the

population under study will benefit from the results;
- Participants must be volunteers and informed in research project;
- Every precaution must be taken to respect privacy, confidentiality, and participant's physical and mental integrity;
- Assent must be obtained from minors, if child able to do so;
- Investigators are obliged to preserve the accuracy of results; negative and positive results should be publicly available.

The Belmont Report (1979)

The Belmont Report, created by the former United States Department of Health, Education and Welfare is an important historical document in the field of medical ethics. The report was created on April 18, 1979 and got its name from the Belmont Conference Center where the document was drafted.

The Belmont Report explains the unifying ethical principles that form the basis for the National Commission's topic-specific reports and the regulations that incorporate its recommendations. The three fundamental ethical principles for using any human subject for research are:

1. Respect for Persons: protecting the autonomy of all people and treating them with courtesy and respect and allowing for informed consent;
2. Beneficence: maximizing benefits for the research project while minimizing risks to the research subjects;
3. Justice: ensuring reasonable, non-exploitative and well considered procedures are administered fairly (the fair distribution of costs and benefits to potential research participants).

The applications of 1, 2, and 3, respectively, are informed consent, assessment of risks and benefits, and selection of subjects.

ICH - Good Clinical Practice (GCP) of 1997

The Food and Drug Administration (FDA) has published guidelines entitled "Good Clinical Practice: Consolidated Guideline". The guideline was prepared under the auspices of the International Conference on Harmonization of Technical Requirements for Registration of Pharmaceuticals for Human Use (ICH). The guideline is intended to define "Good Clinical Practice" and to provide a unified ethical and scientific quality standard for designing, conducting, recording and reporting trials that involve the participation of human subjects. Compliance with this standard provides public assurance that the rights, safety and well being of trial subjects are protected, consistent with the principles that have their origin in the Declaration of Helsinki, and that the clinical trial data are credible.

The objective of the ICH-GCP Guidelines is to provide a unified standard for the European Union (EU), Japan and the United States to facilitate the mutual acceptance of clinical data by the regulatory authorities in these jurisdictions. The guideline was developed with consideration of the current good clinical practices of the European Union, Japan, and the United States, as well as those of Australia, Canada, the Nordic countries and the World Health Organization (WHO). These guidelines are required to be followed while generating clinical trial data that is intended to be submitted to regulatory authorities. The principles established in this guideline may also be applied to other clinical investigations that may have an impact on the safety and well-being of human subjects.

The Principles of GCP

1. Clinical trials should be conducted in accordance with the ethical principles that have their origin in the Declaration of Helsinki, and that are consistent with GCP and the applicable regulatory requirement(s).
2. Before a trial is initiated, foreseeable risks and inconveniences should be weighed against the anticipated benefit for the individual trial subject and society. A trial should be initiated and continued only if the anticipated benefits justify the risks.
3. The rights, safety, and well being of the trial subjects are the most important considerations and should prevail over interests of science and society.
4. The available non-clinical and clinical information on an investigational product should be adequate to support the proposed clinical trial.
5. Clinical trials should be scientifically sound, and describes in a clear, detailed protocol.
6. A trial should be conducted in compliance with the protocol that has received prior institutional review board (IRB)/independent ethics committee (IEC) approval/favourable opinion.
7. The medical care given to, and medical decisions made on behalf of, subjects should always be the responsibility of a qualified physician or, when appropriate, of a qualified dentist.
8. Each individual involved in conducting a trial should be qualified by education, training, and experience to perform his or her respective task(s).
9. Freely given informed consent should be obtained from every subject prior to clinical trial participation.

10. All clinical trial information should be recorded, handled, and stored in a way that allows its accurate reporting, interpretation, and verification.

11. The confidentiality of records that could identify subjects should be protected, respecting the privacy and confidentiality rules in accordance with the applicable regulatory requirement(s).

12. Investigational products should be manufactured, handled, and stored in accordance with applicable good manufacturing practice (GMP). They should be used in accordance with the approved protocol. Systems with procedures that assure the quality of every aspect of the trial should be implemented.

13. System with procedures that assure the quality of every aspect of the trials should be implemented.

3

Essential Clinical Trial Documents

Essential clinical trial documents individually and collectively evaluate the conduct of a trial and preserve the integrity of the data. These are essential to demonstrate the compliance of the investigator and sponsor/CRO with the standards of GCP and all applicable regulatory requirements. Some of the important essential clinical trial documents include:

1. Protocol

A document that states the background, objectives, rationale, design, methodology (including the methods for dealing with AEs, withdrawals *etc.*) and statistical considerations of the study. It also states the conditions under which the study shall be performed and managed.

The term Protocol, unless otherwise specified, relates to the latest amended version of the document, read in conjunction with all its appendices and enclosures. The content and format of the protocol should take into consideration the adopted SOPs, the regulatory requirements and the guiding principles of GCP.

General Tips on Protocol

- Protocol must contain all the ICH-GCP required elements as specified in Section 6.
- A version date and a version number should identify the approved protocol.
- Regulatory and ethics committee approval must be obtained for each clinical trial protocol.
- Version control should be maintained for all subsequent amendments.
- A tracking log should be maintained to record version(s) control.

2. Informed Consent Document (ICD)

A document for voluntary written consent of a subject's willingness to participate in a particular study. The confirmation is sought only after information about the trial including an explanation of its status as research, its objectives, potential benefits, risks and inconveniences, alternative treatment that may be available and of the subject's rights and responsibilities has been provided to the potential subject.

General Tips on ICD

- ICD must contain all the ICH-GCP required elements as specified in Section 4.8.10.
- A version date and a version number should identify each ICD.
- Translation of ICD in vernacular languages must be approved by ethics committee.
- Only the ethics committee approved version of ICD should be administered to the patients.
- Version control should be maintained for all subsequent amendments.
- A tracking log should be maintained to record version(s) control.
- ICD should be obtained before non-routine screening procedures are performed and/or before any change in the subject's current medical therapy is made for the purpose of the clinical trial.
- Investigator or designee should personally obtain the ICD from the subject.
- Subject should receive a copy of the signed ICD.

3. Investigator's Brochure (IB)

A collection of data (including justification for the proposed study) for the Investigator consisting of all the clinical as well as non-clinical information available on the Investigational Product (s) known prior to the onset of the trial. There should be adequate data to justify the nature, scale and duration of the proposed trial and to evaluate the potential safety and need for special precautions. If new substantially relevant data is generated during the trial, the information in the Investigator's Brochure must be updated.

General Tips on IB

- IB must contain all the ICH-GCP required elements as specified in Section 7.
- A version date and a version number should identify each IB.
- Ethics committee must review each version of IB.
- IB should be updated on a regular interval to include all new data on the Investigational product.
- Previous version of IB should be destroyed once the updated version is available.

4. Case Record Form / Clinical Report Form (CRF)

A document designed in consonance with the protocol, to record data and other information on each trial subject. The Case Record Form should be in such a form and format that allows accurate input, presentation, verification, audit and inspection of the recorded data. A CRF may be in printed or electronic format.

General Tips on CRF

- CRF should be designed to include all the required data.
- CRF should preferably be made of NCR (no carbon required) paper.

5. Source Data/Document (SD)

The term source data/document refers to the original documents (or their verified and certified copies) necessary for evaluation of the Clinical Trial. These documents may include Study Subject's files, recordings from automated instruments, tracings, X-Ray and other films, laboratory notes, photographic negatives, magnetic media, hospital records, clinical and office charts, Subject's diaries, evaluation checklists, and pharmacy dispensing records.

General Tips on SD

- All entries in worksheets or patient files should have the date and initials of person making the entry.
- All the records of a patient should be filed in one file or together. If the patient is referred to another department/hospital, all the relevant records should be included in the source document.
- Start and stop date for all adverse event(s) and corrective medication(s) should be clearly stated in the patient's source document.
- Environmental control (protection from fire, flood, termite *etc.*) must be maintained throughout the duration of archival.

6. Regulatory Approval

A document to grant permission for the conduct of a trial at respective investigator site(s) in a country.

General Tips on Regulatory Approval

- Regulatory approval must be obtained prior to initiating any clinical trial.
- Regulatory approval must contain the duration of approval.

7. ERB/IRB/IEC/EC Approval

A document to grant permission for the conduct of a trial at individual investigator site.

General Tips on ERB/IRB/IEC/EC Approval

- ERB approval should include the name and version(s) of the documents reviewed for granting approval.
- ERB approval must contain signature, date and seal of chairperson; list of voting members; and list of members who were absent.
- ERB approval must contain the duration of approval.
- ERB approval must be obtained prior to initiating a clinical trial at any site

8. Advertisement

Advertisement for subject recruitment (if used) is a document that provides brief study outline to recruit the potential patients. It is important to ensure that recruitment measures are appropriate and not coercive.

General Tips on Advertisement

- All trial related advertisement must be approved by ethics committee.
- Wordings of advertisement should be such that it does not coerce the patient(s) to participate in a clinical trial.

9. Financial Agreement

A document to disclose the financial aspect of the trial between the investigator/institution and the sponsor.

General Tips on Financial Agreements

- All trial related financial agreement should be in compliance with the individual institution and the local laws.
- The hospital administration and the ethics committee should be made aware of the financial aspect of the trial.
- All trial related grants/payments should be made in accordance with the financial agreement.

10. Insurance Statement

A document to indemnify that the compensation to subject(s) for trial-related injury will be available.

General Tips on Insurance Statement

- Sponsor should provide the insurance statement prior to initiating the trial at a particular site.

- Insurance statement should include the compensation clause for all trial related injuries.

11. Curriculum Vitae (CV)

A document to provide qualifications and eligibility of investigator(s), sub-investigator(s), co-investigator(s), co-ordinator(s), nurse/pharmacist, sponsor designee(s) and other relevant study personnel.

General Tips on CV

- CV must be obtained from all the concerned personnel prior to initiating a clinical trial.

- CV should be personally signed and dated by the concerned personnel.

12. Laboratory Reference Range

A document containing normal values and/or ranges of the laboratory test at the individual trial site/laboratory.

General Tips on Laboratory Reference Range

- Laboratory reference range must be obtained prior to initiating the clinical trial at a particular site.

- It should be personally signed and dated by the concerned personnel.

13. Monitoring Report

A document prepared by the sponsor's designee on the trial progress at individual trial site(s) after the monitoring/inspection visit.

General Tips on Monitoring Report

- Monitoring report should include all finding and issues with actionable and timelines.

- Monitoring report should document all violations and protocol non-compliance.

14. Investigational Product Accountability Log

A document to provide complete accountability of investigational product including receipt, dispensing, returned, destruction *etc.* at all levels (sponsor, investigator and patient level).

General Tips on Investigational Product Accountability

- Investigational product(s) should be stored at required temperature/ humidity conditions.
- Temperature/humidity logs should be maintained on a daily basis.
- Investigational product should be kept under proper access control.
- Any deviation in storage condition should be reported appropriately and the material should be inspected for potency (if required)
- Reconciliation of all used/unused investigational product(s) should be available at the site(s) and sponsor level.
- Any loss/damage/breakage *etc.* should be properly documented.
- Destruction certificate of investigational product(s) should be available at all levels.

15. Certificate(s) of Analysis (COA)

A document to provide identity, purity and strength of investigational product(s) used in a trial.

General Tips on COA

- COA should be present for each batch and class of investigational product(s).
- COA should be available prior to initiating the clinical trial.

16. SAE Reporting Form

A document or template to report Serious Adverse Event(s) of a trial to the sponsor and the ethics committee.

General Tips on SAE Reporting

- An SAE should be reported only if it meets the requirements of a valid case (*i.e.* an identifiable patient; an identifiable reporter; a suspect drug or biological product; and an adverse event or fatal outcome).
- All the SAEs must meet the reporting timelines as specified by the sponsor.
- All the SAEs and follow-up reports at a particular site should be reported to respective ethics committee.
- All the valid SAE cases should be reported to applicable regulatory

authority(ies) within the stipulated timeframe.

17. Correspondence

Documentation of trial specific communication between various involved parties (sponsor, investigator, ethics committee, regulatory agency *etc*.).

General Tips on Correspondence

- All correspondence should contain a date and an identifiable reporter.
- All correspondence should be filed to provide an audit trail.

18. Queries

Documentation of CRF corrections including all changes/ additions or corrections made to CRF after initial data has been reviewed and collected.

General Tips on Queries

- The designated personnel should sign all queries.
- Individual query should be filed with the respective CRF page for which the query is generated.

19. Clinical Study Report (CSR)

A report prepared at the end of a trial including results and interpretation.

General Tips on CSR

- CSR should be prepared irrespective of the trial outcome (positive or negative).
- CSR should be submitted to applicable regulatory bodies.

4

Clinical Study Process

Clinical Research is a team effort and requires involvement of various stakeholders to achieve the planned endpoint. Each stakeholder has a defined role in the overall clinical study process and the smooth execution of a clinical trial is largely dependent on efficient functioning of individual stakeholder. The various stakeholders include:

- Sponsor(s)/ Contract Research Organizations (CROs)
- Investigator(s)
- EC (Ethics Committee)
- Regulatory Authorities (*e.g.* US-FDA, MHRA, EMEA, TGA *etc.*)
- Patients/Study Subjects

Figure 3 represents association of various stakeholders in the overall clinical study process.

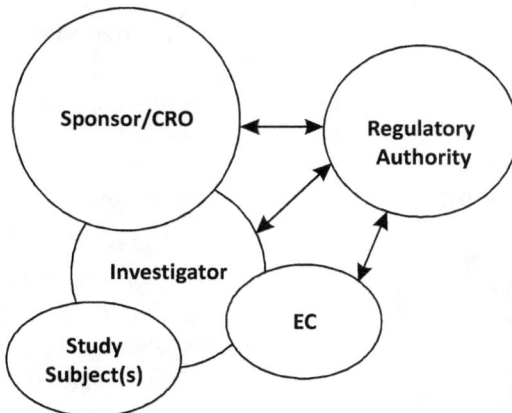

Figure 3: Clinical Trial Stakeholders

The chief responsibilities of individual stakeholder are as follows:

Sl. No.	Stakeholder	Chief Responsibility(ies)
1.	Sponsor/CRO	- Trial planning and allocation of resources - Financial and milestones planning - Selection and training of investigators, monitors and study staff - Regulatory approval and trial conduct - Data monitoring and management - Compliance with GCP and applicable regulatory guidelines - Auditing and QA - Publication of trial results
2.	Investigator	- Constitution and training of study team at the site - Obtaining ethics approval for the study - Study conduct/enrolment of study subjects - Medical care of study subjects and safety reporting - Compliance with GCP and applicable regulatory guidelines
3.	ERB/IRB/IEC	- Trial permission/approval - Review of trial progress - Trial termination/suspension - Compliance with GCP and applicable regulatory guidelines - Inspection of study site
4.	Regulatory Authority	- Trial permission/approval - Review of trial progress - Trial termination/suspension

Sl. No.	Stakeholder	Chief Responsibility(ies)
		- Implementation of GCP and applicable regulatory guidelines - Inspection of sponsor, CRO, investigator, ERB/IRB/IEC *etc.*
5.	Study Subject	- Voluntary participation in the trial and ensuring compliance with protocol schedule of events

Clinical study process involves the participation of individual stakeholder for the responsibilities mentioned above during following stages:

1. Initiating a Clinical Trial
2. Conduct of the Trial
3. Trial Closure
4. Registration/Publication

Clinical Study Process Part 1: Initiating a Clinical Trial

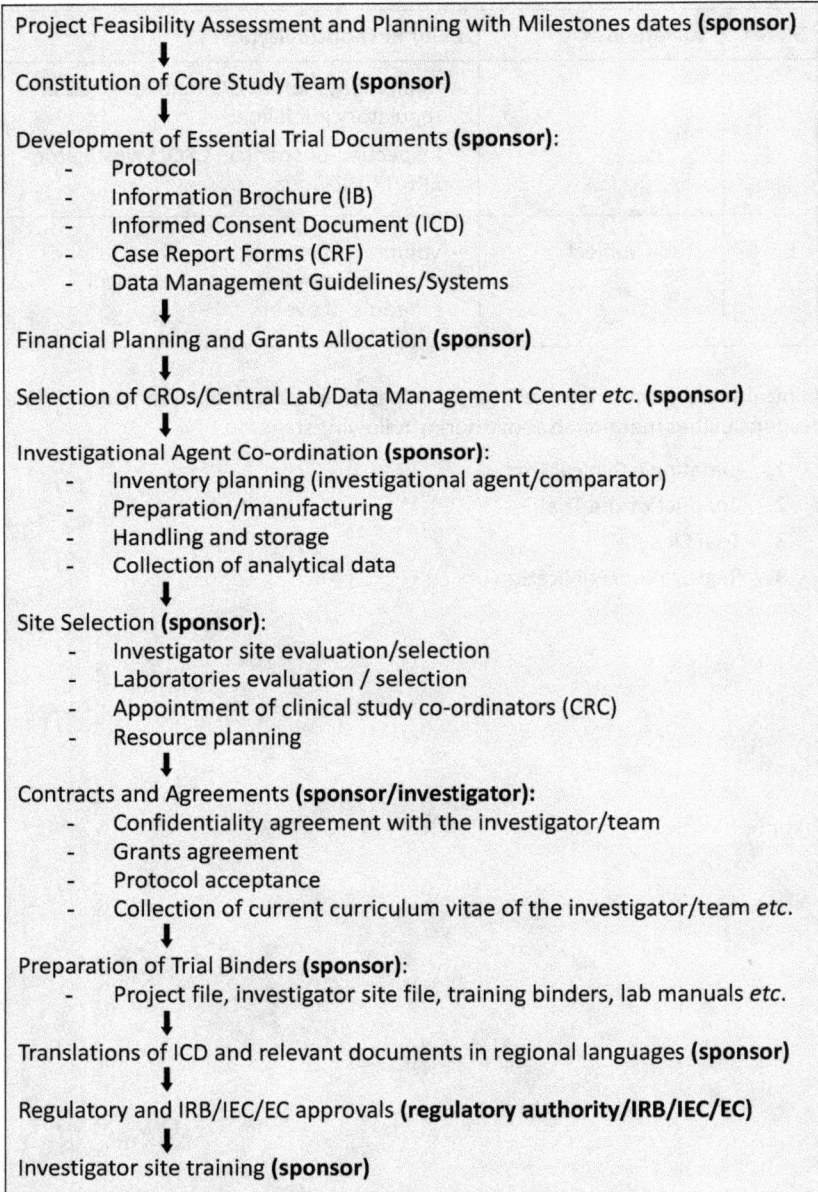

Project Feasibility Assessment and Planning with Milestones dates **(sponsor)**
↓
Constitution of Core Study Team **(sponsor)**
↓
Development of Essential Trial Documents **(sponsor)**:
- Protocol
- Information Brochure (IB)
- Informed Consent Document (ICD)
- Case Report Forms (CRF)
- Data Management Guidelines/Systems

↓
Financial Planning and Grants Allocation **(sponsor)**
↓
Selection of CROs/Central Lab/Data Management Center *etc.* **(sponsor)**
↓
Investigational Agent Co-ordination **(sponsor)**:
- Inventory planning (investigational agent/comparator)
- Preparation/manufacturing
- Handling and storage
- Collection of analytical data

↓
Site Selection **(sponsor)**:
- Investigator site evaluation/selection
- Laboratories evaluation / selection
- Appointment of clinical study co-ordinators (CRC)
- Resource planning

↓
Contracts and Agreements **(sponsor/investigator)**:
- Confidentiality agreement with the investigator/team
- Grants agreement
- Protocol acceptance
- Collection of current curriculum vitae of the investigator/team *etc.*

↓
Preparation of Trial Binders **(sponsor)**:
- Project file, investigator site file, training binders, lab manuals *etc.*

↓
Translations of ICD and relevant documents in regional languages **(sponsor)**
↓
Regulatory and IRB/IEC/EC approvals **(regulatory authority/IRB/IEC/EC)**
↓
Investigator site training **(sponsor)**

Note : Sponsor can delegate part or all of its responsibilities to a CRO

Clinical Study Process Part 2: Conduct of the Trial

Study Initiation **(sponsor/CRO)**
↓
Trial Conduct **(investigator):**
- Delegation of duties at the site
- Administration of ICD
- Recruitment of study subjects
- Administration of investigational product/comparator
- Medical care of study subjects
- Data collection and management
- Management and reporting of AEs/SAEs
- Compliance with protocol schedule of events
- Compliance with ICH-GCP and applicable regulatory guidelines

↓
Participation in the Trial **(patient/study subject):**
- Voluntary consent and compliance with protocol schedule of events

↓
Monitoring of Trial to ensure **(sponsor/CRO):**
- Protocol, GCP and regulatory compliance, drug accountability, audit trail, data collection, good documentation

↓
Overall Site Management **(investigator/sponsor/CRO)**
↓
Management of Logistics and Clinical Trial Supplies **(sponsor/CRO/ investigator)**
↓
Adverse Events Recording and Reporting **(investigator/sponsor/CRO)**
↓
Ongoing Data Management **(sponsor/CRO)**
↓
Periodic Reporting to IRB/IEC/EC **(investigator)**
↓
Periodic Reporting to Regulatory Agencies **(sponsor/CRO)**
↓
Meeting the Project Timelines **(sponsor/CRO/investigator)**
↓
Payments as per Schedule **(sponsor/CRO)**
↓
Amendment(s) to the Study if required **(sponsor/CRO)**
↓
Quality Assurance **(sponsor/CRO)**
↓
Ongoing Training and Development for new/existing staff **(sponsor/CRO)**

Note : Sponsor can delegate part or all of its responsibilities to a CRO

Clinical Study Process Part 3: Trial Closure

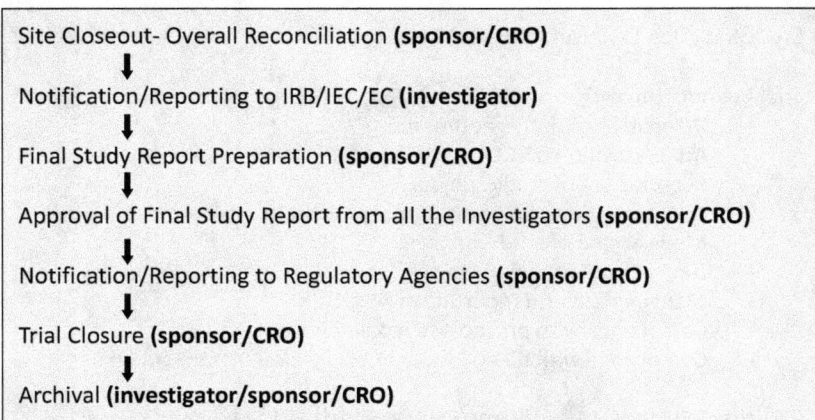

Site Closeout- Overall Reconciliation **(sponsor/CRO)**
↓
Notification/Reporting to IRB/IEC/EC **(investigator)**
↓
Final Study Report Preparation **(sponsor/CRO)**
↓
Approval of Final Study Report from all the Investigators **(sponsor/CRO)**
↓
Notification/Reporting to Regulatory Agencies **(sponsor/CRO)**
↓
Trial Closure **(sponsor/CRO)**
↓
Archival **(investigator/sponsor/CRO)**

Note : Sponsor can delegate part or all of its responsibilities to a CRO

Clinical Study Process Part 4: Registration/Publication

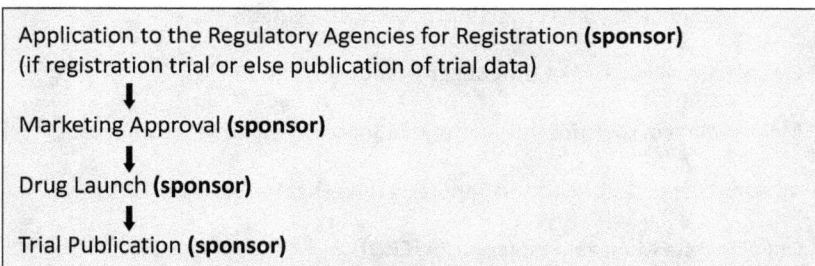

Application to the Regulatory Agencies for Registration **(sponsor)**
(if registration trial or else publication of trial data)
↓
Marketing Approval **(sponsor)**
↓
Drug Launch **(sponsor)**
↓
Trial Publication **(sponsor)**

5

Ethics Review Board (ERB)

Ethics Review Board is an independent body constituted of medical/scientific professionals and non-medical/non-scientific members, whose responsibility is to ensure the protection of rights, safety and well being of human subjects involved in a trial. ERB ensures a competent review of all the ethical aspects of the project proposals received and executes the same free from any bias and influence that could affect their objectivity. It might have different names at different institutions but the prime responsibility remains the same. ERB is also known as:

- Independent Ethics Committee (IEC)
- Institutional Review Board (IRB)
- Ethics Committee (EC)

The main responsibilities of ERB are:

- to safeguard the dignity, rights, safety and well being of the potential research participants.
- to ensure and verify that universal ethical values and international scientific standards are followed with a view on local community values and customs.

Composition of ERB

The ERB usually consists of a reasonable number of members, who collectively have the qualification and experience to review and evaluate the science, medical aspects and ethics of the proposed trial. An ideal ERB should include (as per ICH-GCP, 1997) :

- At least five members (quorum).
- At least one member whose primary area of interest is in non-scientific area.
- At least one member who is independent of the institution/trial site.

ERB Charter

The charter of ERB should be defined in its written standard operating procedures (SOP).

It is recommended that the ERB should:

- maintain records of its activities and minutes of its meetings.
- comply with ICH-GCP and applicable regulatory requirement(s).
- makes its decision at announced meetings (at which at least a quorum), as stipulated in the operating procedures, is present.
- include only those members who are independent of the investigator and of the trial in the voting process.
- include only those members in the voting process who are present during the review meeting.

ERB Responsibilities

1. Approval/Permission for the Conduct of Clinical Trials

No clinical trial should be initiated at any investigator site without obtaining a written approval/permission of the essential trial documents from the respective ERB. An Independent Ethics Committee can be approached if the investigator site does not have an ERB of its own. Following documents requires ERB review and approval before initiating a clinical trial at a site:

- study protocol.
- patient information sheet (PIS) and informed consent form (ICF).
- translations of PIS and ICF in vernacular languages along with the translation validation certificates.
- investigator's brochure (IB) for all relevant clinical and non-clinical data on investigational product.
- undertaking by the investigator along with recent curriculum vitae.
- insurance/indemnity certificate(s).
- clinical trial agreement (CTA).
- subject recruitment procedures (*e.g.* advertisements if applicable).
- any other written information to be provided to the subjects (*e.g.* patient diaries/cards, questionnaires *etc.*).
- regulatory approval of the trial.

2. Review of Progress

After granting the approval for the conduct of clinical trial(s) it is the responsibility of ERB to have an ongoing review of the trial progress. This include:

- review of safety reports (reports of serious adverse events).
- review and approval of the amendment(s) if applicable.
- review of protocol/process deviations or violations.

The frequency of these reviews may vary across institutions however it should be clearly stated in the Standard Operating Procedure (SOP) of the ERB .

3. Compliance with the Regulatory Requirements

In order to ensure regulatory compliance each ERB is required to maintain following records:

- written standard operating procedures or charter.
- constitution and composition as stipulated in the guidelines.
- curriculum vitae of all ERB members.
- copies of all the trial(s) documents received for review.
- all the correspondence betweenERB and investigator.
- agenda and minutes of all ERB meetings.
- final report of the study.

The review should be done through formal meetings and should not resort to decisions through circulation of proposals.

Examples of Violations at the Level of ERB

- failure to fulfill expedited review requirements.
- inadequate documentation of ERB activities.
    - poor minutes
    - poor records of communication with investigator
- undocumented or non-existent training for members and/or staff.
- failure to conduct adequate review :
    - absence of a member from outside the institution.
    - failure to ensure that research is free of conflict of interests.
    - review without a majority of voting members being present.
    - inadequate review of adverse events.
    - inadequate review of patient recruitment advertisements *etc.*

6

Roles and Responsibilities of Investigator

Investigator is a person responsible for the conduct of clinical trial at a trial site. If a trial is conducted by a team of individuals at a site, the investigator is the responsible leader of the team and may be called as principal investigator. Sub-investigator is any individual member of the clinical trial team designated and supervised by the investigator to perform critical trial-related procedures and/or to make important trial-related decisions (*e.g.*, associates, residents, research fellows).

FDA regulations (21CFR 312.52) and ICH Guidelines (ICH 4.1) mandates that sponsors works with trained and qualified investigators.

Responsibilities of Investigator

1. **Initiating a Clinical Trial**

   a. **Contracts and agreements**: Investigator is responsible to enter into trial related agreements as per applicable regulatory requirements *i.e.* confidentiality agreement, protocol/trial acceptance, roles and responsibilities delegation, grants and payments agreements *etc.*

   b **Obtaining ERB/IEC/IRB approval**: It is the responsibility of investigator to obtain ERB approval of the study and to ensure that the patient enrolment in the study begins only after such approval.

   c. **Constitution of study team**: It is the responsibility of investigator to constitute a study team including co-investigator(s), sub-investigator(s), clinical research coordinator(s), study nurse/pharmacist *etc.* for the smooth execution of a clinical trial.

   d. **Allocation of resources required for the conduct of a trial**: The investigator is responsible to ensure the availability of adequate facilities at the site as per the specific requirements of a clinical trial.

   e. **Participation in the investigator training meeting**: The investigator is responsible to ensure that he/she and all of his/her team members attends the investigator training meeting organized by the sponsor of the study.

2. Conduct of the Trial

a. Recruitment/Enrolment of the subjects in the study:

i. Investigator is responsible for the unbiased selection of eligible subjects for enrolment into the study. If required, he/she may seek the co-operation of other physicians to recruit the required number of subjects.

ii. Investigator is responsible for maintaining the subject identification log as well as subject screening/enrolment log to document the identification as well as enrolment of the study subjects.

b. Informed Consent Document (ICD) administration:

i. The investigator is responsible for ensuring the compliance with the applicable regulatory requirement(s), in obtaining and documenting the informed consent from the study subject(s).

ii. It is the responsibility of the investigator to ensure that ICD has been approved by ERB/IRB/IEC and the same has been revised and re-approved whenever important new information becomes available that may be relevant to the subject's decision to continue participation in the study.

iii. Investigator is responsible to ensure that neither he/she, nor any of the trial staff, is coercing or unduly influencing a subject to participate or to continue to participate in a trial.

iv. It is the responsibility of investigator to provide clear oral and written information about the trial in a language most easily understandable by subject or his/her legal representative.

v. It is the responsibility of investigator to ensure that ample time and opportunity to inquire about details of the trial and to decide whether or not to participate in the trial is provided to the subject or the subject's legally acceptable representative, before obtaining the informed consent.

vi. Investigator is responsible to ensure that the written informed consent form has been signed and dated by the subject or his/her legally acceptable representative (or by an impartial witness in case subject or his/her legally acceptable representative is unable to read), and by the person who conducted the informed consent discussion/documentation prior to a subject's participation in the trial.

vii. Investigator is responsible to ensure that both the informed consent discussion and the written informed consent form or any other written information provided to the subject(s) clearly explains the purpose of the trial, the trial treatment(s) and the probability for random assignment to the treatment (if applicable), the trial procedures to be followed (experimental/non experimental), including all invasive procedures, the subject's responsibilities, the foreseeable risks or inconveniences and expected benefits, the alternative procedure(s) or course(s) of treatment options that may be available to the subject with their benefits and risks, the compensation and/or treatment available to the subject in the event of trial-related injury and voluntary nature of the subject's participation in the trial *etc.*

viii. Investigator is responsible to ensure that the confidentiality and identity of subjects and their records is protected during the trial related publications/regulatory submissions.

c. **Medical care of the trial subjects**: The investigator is responsible for the appropriate medical care of the trial subject and of ensuring that adequate medical care is provided to a subject for any adverse event, including clinically significant laboratory values during subject's participation in a trial.

d. **Compliance with protocol schedule of events**: The investigator is responsible to comply with the protocol schedule of events and of ensuring that no deviation or changes to the protocol is implemented without the agreement of the sponsor and prior review and documented approval of the ERB/IRB/IEC, except where necessary to eliminate an immediate hazard(s) to trial subjects, or when the change(s) involves only logistical or administrative aspects of the trial (*e.g.*, change in monitor, change of telephone number *etc.*).

e. **Compliance with ICH-GCP/applicable regulatory requirements**: It is the responsibility of investigator to comply with, GCP and the applicable regulatory requirement at all times.

f. **Investigational product(s) storage, handling and accountability**:

   i. The investigator is responsible for obtaining the training on the appropriate use of the investigational product(s), as per the the protocol/investigator's brochure.

   ii. The investigator is responsible for maintaining the accountability of investigational product(s) at the trial site.

   iii. The investigator is responsible for maintaining the records of investigational product(s) administration (dose/interval) to the subjects as well as the temperature logs for its appropriate storage condition.

g. **Randomization procedures and unblinding**: Where applicable an investigator is responsible to follow the randomization and unblinding procedures as specified by the sponsor.

h. **Communication with ERB/IRB/IEC**: The investigator is responsible for submitting the ongoing safety updates, progress reports, amendment to the study documents (if applicable) to the ERB/IRB/IEC annually, or more frequently, if required by applicable authority(ies).

i. **Communication with sponsor (enrolment, randomization, safety reporting** *etc.***)**:

   i. The investigator is responsible to immediately report all serious adverse events (SAEs) to the sponsor followed promptly by detailed, written reports except for those SAEs that the protocol or other document (*e.g.*, Investigator's Brochure) identifies as not needing immediate reporting requirements.

   ii. The investigator is responsible to comply with the applicable regulatory requirement(s) related to the reporting of unexpected serious adverse drug reactions to the regulatory authority(ies) and the ERB/IRB/IEC.

   iii. The investigator is responsible to make all other trial related communications like enrolment updates, randomization details, unblinding *etc.* as per the specification of the sponsor.

j. **Facilitating data collection and monitoring**: The investigator is responsible to ensure the accuracy, completeness, legibility, and timeliness of the data reported in the CRFs and in all required reports.

k. **Documenting errors, violations, non-compliance** *etc.* and taking appropriate actions to avoid them in future.

l. **Financial tracking:** The investigator is responsible for maintaining the records of payments made to trial staff or to subjects (if any) and of other trial related expenses.

m. **Ensuring confidentiality** of trial subjects and integrity of trial data throughout the course of trial and thereafter as recommended.

n. **Facilitating the site audit** (if any).

3. **Site Closure**

   a. **Final report to ERB/IRB/IEC**: Upon completion of the trial, it is the responsibility of the investigator, where applicable, to report a summary on the outcome of the trial to the ERB/IRB/IEC.

   b. **Providing all data/documents required at site closure to Sponsor.**

   c. **Return of equipment (if any) and investigational product (both used and unused) as well as reconcilation of the study grants.**

   d. **Archival of trial data for the duration specified in the contract**: The investigator is responsible to ensure the archival of all trial related essential documents as per the applicable regulatory requirements or as per the agreement with the sponsor.

   e. **Premature termination or suspension of a trial**: In case of premature suspension/termination of a trial for any reason, it is the responsibility of the investigator to promptly inform the trial subjects, and to take care for the appropriate therapy and follow-up of the subjects. In case the investigator terminates or suspends a trial without prior agreement of the sponsor, he/she should inform the institution/sponsor/ ERB/IRB/IEC with a detailed written explanation for the termination or suspension.

7

Roles and Responsibilities of Sponsor

Sponsor is an individual, company, institution or organization which takes responsibility for the initiation, management and/or financing of a clinical trial.

Responsibilities of Sponsor

1. Investigator and Institution /Hospital (Site) Selection

a. It is the responsibility of sponsor to select well qualified, trained and experienced investigator(s) for the conduct of the trial. The selected investigator should be based at the institutions/hospitals having sufficient resources to properly conduct the trial.

b. Sponsor is responsible to provide a copy of the protocol and an up-to-date investigator's brochure to the investigator(s) and give them a sufficient time for the review of the study documents.

2. Contract/Agreements

It is the responsibility of sponsor to enter into an agreement with the investigator/ institution for the conduct of the trial according to the GCP and applicable regulatory requirements. The agreement should clearly define:

a. that the trial would be conducted in compliance with the protocol provided by the sponsor and approved by the ERB/IRB/IEC.

b. that sponsor's Standard Operating Procedures (SOPs) for data recording/ reporting/conduct of trial would be followed.

c. that sponsor has the right to monitor, audit and inspect site at any time.

d. that investigator(s)/Institution(s) have to retain the trial related essential documents for the duration defined by appropriate regulatory bodies or until the sponsor's specifications.

e. that funding of the trial *i.e* financial support, fees, honorarium will be provided by the sponsor

3. Duties and Functions Allocation

The sponsor is responsible to identify, define and allocate all trial-related functions and duties to the qualified person (s)/organization(s)/ institution(s)

before the initiation of a trial.

4. Clinical Trial Management, Data Handling and Record Keeping

a. It is the responsibility of sponsor to select the qualified individuals to supervise the overall conduct of the trial, to handle the data, to verify the data, to conduct the statistical analyses, and to prepare the trial reports.

b. Sponsor is responsible to establish an independent data-monitoring committee (IDMC) to assess the progress of a clinical trial, including the safety and efficacy data, and to recommend to the sponsor whether to continue, modify, or stop a trial.

c. It is the responsibility of sponsor to meet the applicable standards for completeness, accuracy, reliability and consistency of the data processing systems for electronic trial data handling systems.

d. Sponsor is responsible for maintaining the sponsor-specific essential documents in conformance with the applicable regulatory requirement(s).

e. Sponsor is responsible to report to the appropriate regulatory body(s)/authority(s) if any transfer of ownership of the clinical data takes place.

f. Sponsor is responsible for maintaining the data confidentiality as per applicable guidelines (*i.e* HIPAA guidelines).

g. the sponsor is responsible to place appropriate quality assurance and quality control systems with written SOPs to ensure that the study is conducted and data is generated, documented (recorded), and reported in compliance with the Protocol, GCP and the applicable regulatory requirements.

h. Sponsor is responsible for submission of required application(s) to the applicable authority(ies) for the review, acceptance, and/or permission to begin the clinical trial(s). Any notification/submission should be dated and should contain sufficient information to identify the protocol.

5. Compensation to Subjects and Investigators

a. Sponsor is responsible to provide insurance or indemnification (legal and financial coverage) to the investigator/institution, against claims arising from the trial, as per applicable regulatory requirement(s), except for claims that arise from malpractice and/or negligence at the level of investigator/institution.

b. It is the responsibility of sponsor to provide compensation to the trial subjects in accordance with the applicable regulatory requirements.

6. Confirmation of Review by ERB/IRB/IEC

a. Sponsor is responsible for obtaining the name and address of the investigator's/institution's ERB/IRB/IEC, it's SOP, list of members with contact details and qualifications *etc.*

b. Sponsor is responsible for ensuring that ERB/IRB/IEC has reviewed the latest / amended version of protocol, written informed consent form(s) and any other written information to be provided to subjects, subject recruitment procedures, documents related to payments and compensation available to the subjects, and any other documents that the ERB/IRB/IEC may have requested.

c. Sponsor shall ensure that ERB/IRB/IEC approval has been obtained prior to enrolment of any patient in the trial.

7. Information on Investigational Product(s)/Drug(s)

a. Sponsor is responsible to ensure that sufficient safety and efficacy data from non-clinical studies (*i.e.* animal pharmacology and toxicology studies) and/or clinical trials is available for the investigational product/drug to support human exposure.

b. Sponsor is responsible for the review of investigator's brochure at least on an annual basis and revise the same as and when any new information becomes available.

8. Manufacturing, Packaging, Labeling and Coding of Investigational Product(s)

a. Sponsor is responsible to ensure that the investigational product(s) (including active comparator(s) and placebo, if applicable) is manufactured in accordance with applicable regulatory requirements (*e.g.* GMP).

b. Sponsor is responsible to ensure that the investigational product(s) is coded and labeled as per the applicable regulatory requirements.

c. Sponsor is responsible to determine the acceptable storage conditions for the investigational product and of ensuring that all involved parties (*e.g.*, monitors, investigators, pharmacists, storage managers) are aware of these requirements.

d. Sponsor is responsible for suitable packaging of the investigational product in order to prevent the contamination and unacceptable deterioration during transport and storage.

e. Sponsor is responsible to develop a mechanism which permits rapid identification of the investigational product(s) in case of a medical emergency, but does not permit undetectable breaks of the blinding in blinded trials.

9. Supplying and Handling of Investigational Product(s)

a. Sponsor is responsible for supplying the investigational product(s) to all the investigator(s)/institution(s) involved in the trial. The sponsor should not supply the investigational product(s) to an investigator/ institution until the sponsor obtains all required documentation [*e.g.*, approval/favourable opinion from ERB/IRB/IEC and regulatory authority(ies)].

b. Sponsor is responsible for framing and implementing the SOPs for the handling and storage of investigational product(s). The procedures should address adequate and safe receipt, handling, storage, dispensing, retrieval of unused product from subjects, and return of unused investigational product(s) to the sponsor (or disposition if authorized by the sponsor).

c. Sponsor is responsible to retain the samples of the investigational product(s) to the extent stability permits, either until the analyses of the trial data is complete or as required by the applicable regulatory requirement(s), whichever represents the longer retention period.

10. Safety Information

The sponsor is responsible for the ongoing safety evaluation of the investigational product(s). The sponsor should promptly notify all concerned investigator(s)/ institution(s) and the regulatory authority(ies) of findings that could adversely affect the safety of subjects, impact the conduct of the trial, or alter the ERB/IRB/IEC's approval/favourable opinion to continue the trial. The sponsor, together with investigator(s), should take appropriate measures necessary to safeguard the study subjects.

11. Adverse Drug Reaction Reporting

a. Sponsor is responsible for reporting the adverse drug reactions (ADRs) that are both serious and unexpected to all concerned investigator(s)/ institution(s)/IRB(s)/IEC(s) and to the regulatory authority(ies). All such reports/ safety updates should be expedited by the sponsor and should comply with the applicable regulatory requirement(s).

b. Sponsor is responsible to provide a pre-designed ADR/AE reporting form to all the investigator(s).

c. Sponsor is responsible to appoint appropriately qualified medical personnel to advise on trial related medical questions or problems. If required, consultant(s) may be hired for this purpose.

12. Contract Research Organization (CRO) Management

Sponsor may transfer any or all of the sponsor's trial-related duties and functions to a CRO with an agreement in writing, but the ultimate responsibility for the quality and integrity of the trial data always resides with the sponsor. All responsibilities of a sponsor in applicable guideline(s) are also applicable to a CRO to the extent that a CRO has assumed the trial related duties and functions of a sponsor.

13. Record Access

Sponsor is required to have a direct access to the source data/documents for trial-related monitoring, audits, ERB/IRB/IEC review, and regulatory inspection as specified in the protocol or other written agreement with the investigator(s)/institution(s). The sponsor is responsible to verify that each subject has consented in writing for this access.

14. Monitoring

a. It is the responsibility of sponsor to ensure that a clinical trial is adequately monitored. The sponsor should determine the extent and nature of monitoring. The determination of the extent and nature of monitoring should be based on considerations such as the objective, purpose, design, complexity, blinding, size, and endpoints of the trial.

b. Sponsor is responsible for the appointment of monitor to verify the conduct of the trial in compliance with the GCP, protocol and applicable regulatory requirement(s).

15. Audit

a. Sponsor may perform an audit at any or all the trial sites. The purpose of a sponsor's audit, is to evaluate the conduct of the trial as well as compliance with the protocol, SOPs, GCP, and the applicable regulatory requirements.

b. It is the responsibility of sponsor to appoint individuals qualified by training and experience as auditors, who are independent of the clinical trials/systems.

c. It is the responsibility of sponsor to verify the observations and findings of the auditor(s).

d. It is the responsibility of sponsor to provide an audit certificate whenever required by the applicable law or regulation(s).

e. Sponsor is responsible for terminating the participation of a site in the study if monitoring/auditing identify serious and/or persistent non-compliance and promptly notify it to the regulatory authority(ies).

16. Premature Termination or Suspension of a Trial

In case a sponsor choose to or is required to prematurely terminate or suspend a trial, then it's the responsibility of sponsor to promptly inform the investigators/institutions/IRBs/regulatory authority(ies) of the termination or suspension and the reason(s) for the termination or suspension.

17.Clinical Trial/Study Reports

On completion or prematurely termination of the trial, the sponsor is responsible to ensure that the clinical trial reports are prepared and provided to the regulatory agency(ies) as required by the applicable regulatory requirement(s).

18. Multi-centre Trials

a. For multi-centre trials, the sponsor is responsible to ensure that all investigators conduct the trial in strict adherence with the protocol and applicable GCP guidelines.

b. Sponsor is responsible to design the CRFs so as to capture the required data at all multi-centre sites. Supplemental CRFs should be provided to those investigators who are collecting additional data.

c. It is the responsibility of sponsor to ensure that all investigators are given instructions to comply with a uniform set of standards for the protocol, assessment of clinical and laboratory findings, and on completing the CRFs.

d. Sponsor shall try to start and end the study simultaneously at all the institutions.

Chief Responsibilities of the Clinical Trial(s) Sponsor

1. Initiating a Clinical Trial

- Project milestones planning.
- Trial design: development of protocol, information brochure (IB), informed consent document (ICD), case report forms (CRF), data management guidelines/systems.
- Financial planning and grants allocation.
- Investigational agent co-ordination: inventory planning (investigational agent/comparator), handling and storage, preparation, collection of analytical data.
- Site selection: investigator site selection, laboratories selection/ development, clinical study co-ordinators (CRC) appointment, resource planning.
- Contracts and agreements: confidentiality agreement with the investigator/ team, grants agreement, protocol acceptance, collection of updated curriculum vitae of the investigator/ team *etc.*
- Preparation of trial binders: project file, investigator site file, training binders, lab manuals *etc.*
- Translations of ICD and relevant documents in regional languages.
- Regulatory and ERB/IRB/IEC approvals.
- Investigator site training.

2. Conduct of the Trial

- Study initiation.
- Monitoring of trial to ensure protocol compliance, drug accountability, GCP and regulatory compliance.
- Overall site management.
- Management of logistics and clinical trial supplies.
- Adverse events recording and reporting.
- Ongoing data management.
- Periodic reporting to regulatory agencies and ERB.
- Meeting the project timelines.
- Payments of study grants as per schedule.
- Amendment(s) to the study documents (if required).
- Quality assurance.
- Ongoing training and development (for new/existing staff).

3. Trial Closure

- Site closeout and overall reconciliation.
- Notification/reporting to ERB and regulatory agencies.
- Final study report preparation.
- Approval of final study report from all the investigators.
- Trial file closure.
- Archival.

4. Registration/Publication

- Application to the regulatory agencies for registration (if registration trial).
- Publication in peer reviewed journals.
- Marketing approval (if applicable).
- Drug launch (if applicable).

8

Informed Consent

According to ICH-GCP Guidelines, Informed Consent is a process by which a subject voluntarily confirms his or her willingness to participate in a particular trial, after having been informed of all aspects of trial that are relevant to the subject's decision to participate. Informed Consent is documented by means of a written, signed, and dated informed consent document (ICD).

The ICD is used to explain the risks and benefits of study participation to the subject in simple terms and vernacular language, before the subject participates in the study.

ICH-GCP Required Elements for ICD

Sl. No.	ICH Section	Statement
1.	4.8.10 (a)	Trial involves research.
2.	4.8.10 (b)	Purpose of the trial (study objectives).
3.	4.8.10 (c)	Trial treatment and probability for random assignment to each treatment.
4.	4.8.10 (d)	Trial procedures to be followed, including all invasive procedures.
5.	4.8.10 (e)	The subject's responsibilities.
6.	4.8.10 (f)	Aspects of the trial that are experimental.
7.	4.8.10 (g)	The reasonably foreseeable risks or inconvenience to the subject and, when applicable, to an embryo, fetus, or nursing infant.
8.	4.8.10 (h)	The reasonably expected benefits. When there is no intended clinical benefit to the subject, the subject should be made aware of this.

9.	4.8.10(i)	The alternative procedure(s) or course(s) of treatment that may be available to the subject, and their important potential benefits and risks.
10.	4.8.10(j)	The compensation and/or treatment available to the subject in the event of a trial-related injury.
11.	4.8.10(k)	Anticipated prorated payment, if any, to the subject for participating in the trial.
12.	4.8.10(l)	Anticipated expenses, if any, to the subject for participating in the trial.
13.	4.8.10(m)	That the subject's participation in the trial is voluntary and that the subject may refuse to participate or withdraw from the trial, at any time, without penalty or loss of benefits to which the subject is otherwise entitled.
14.	4.8.10(n)	That the monitor(s), the auditor(s), the IRB/IEC, and the regulatory authority(ies) will be granted direct access to the subject's original medical records for verification of clinical trial procedures and/or data, without violating the confidentiality of the subject, to the extent permitted by the applicable laws and regulations and that, by signing a written informed consent form, the subject or the subject's legally acceptable representative is authorizing such access.
15.	4.8.10(o)	That the records identifying the subject will be kept confidential and, to the extent permitted by the applicable laws and/or regulations, will not be made publicly available. If the results of the trial are published, the subject's identity will remain confidential.
16.	4.8.10(p)	That the subject or the subject's legally acceptable representative will be informed in a timely manner if information becomes available that may be relevant to the subject's willingness to continue participation in the trial.
17.	4.8.10(q)	The person(s) to contact for further information regarding the trial and the rights of the trial subjects, and whom to contact in the event of trial-related injury.

18.	4.8.10 (r)	The foreseeable circumstances and/or reasons under which the subject's participation in the trial may be terminated.
19.	4.8.10 (s)	The expected duration of the subject's participation in the trial.
20.	4.8.10 (t)	The approximate number of subjects involved in the trial.

Requirements for obtaining Informed Consent in a Clinical Trial:

- The investigator, or a person knowledgeable about the trial and designated by the investigator, must obtain informed consent.

- Informed Consent must be obtained before non-routine screening procedures are performed and/or before any change in the subject's current medical therapy is made for the purpose of the clinical trial.

- The subject (or legally acceptable representative*) should have ample opportunity to ask questions and to decide whether or not to participate in the clinical trial.

- The subject should not be coerced to participate or continue to participate in a trial.

- The subject (or legally acceptable representative) and the individual obtaining consent must personally sign and date (with the time, where appropriate) the ICD.

- The signature of the prospective subject or legally acceptable representative on the ICD indicates that the content of the ICD has been adequately discussed, and the subject or legally acceptable representative freely gave that informed consent.

- The subject or legally acceptable representative should receive a copy of the signed ICD and any subsequent amendments.

- In situation where the subject can be enrolled in a trial only with the consent of a legally acceptable representative, (*e.g.* minors, or subjects with severe dementia), the subject should still be informed of the clinical trial compatible with the subject's level of understanding. In addition to the legally acceptable representative, the subject should (if capable) personally sign and date (with time, if appropriate) the ICD (or other equivalent document) following an explanation of the clinical trial.

* An individual or juridical or other body authorized under applicable law to consent, on behalf of a prospective subject, to the subject's participation in the clinical trial.

Special Circumstances:

- In emergency situations, when prior consent of the subject is not possible, the consent of the subject's legally acceptable representative, if present, should be requested.

- When prior consent of the subject is not possible, and the subject's legally acceptable representative is unable to be physically present to read and sign the ICD, or a legally acceptable representative is not available, enrolment of the subject should require measures described in the protocol and/or elsewhere, with documented approval/favorable opinion by the IRB/IEC, to protect the rights, safety and well-being of the subject and to ensure compliance with applicable regulatory requirements. The subject or the subject's legally acceptable representative should be informed about the trial as soon as possible and consent to continue and other consent as appropriate should be requested.

- In situations where the subject or legally acceptable representative is unable to read, an impartial witness** should be present during the informed consent discussions. After oral consent has been obtained from the subject or legally acceptable representative, and after the subject or legally acceptable representative has signed and dated the ICD (if he/she is capable of doing so), the witness should also sign and date the ICD. This signature and date indicates that the information in the consent form was accurately explained to the subject or legally acceptable representative and the subject or legally acceptable representative freely gave that informed consent.

**A person, who is independent of the trial, who cannot be unfairly influenced by the people involved with the trial, who attends the informed consent process if the subject or the subject's legally acceptable representative cannot read, and who reads the informed consent form and any other written information supplied to the subject.

Process Flow for obtaining Informed Consent Document from Literates

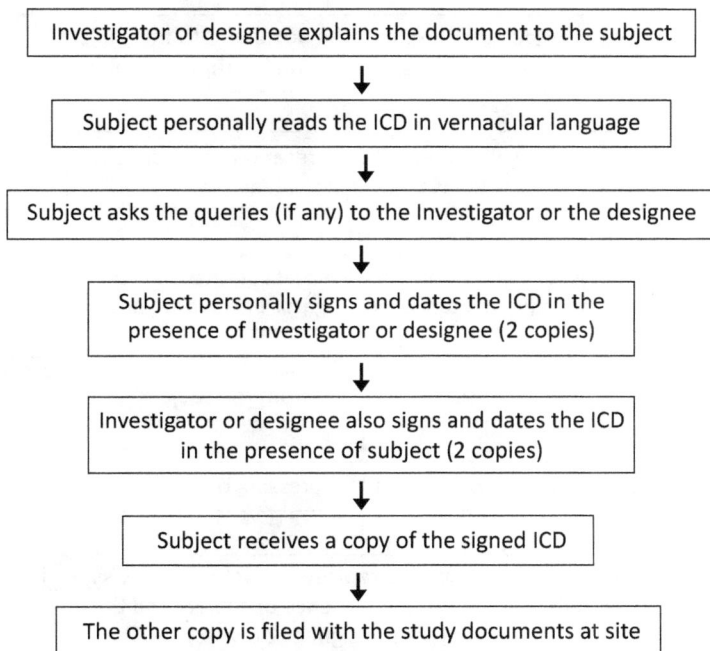

Investigator or designee explains the document to the subject

↓

Subject personally reads the ICD in vernacular language

↓

Subject asks the queries (if any) to the Investigator or the designee

↓

Subject personally signs and dates the ICD in the presence of Investigator or designee (2 copies)

↓

Investigator or designee also signs and dates the ICD in the presence of subject (2 copies)

↓

Subject receives a copy of the signed ICD

↓

The other copy is filed with the study documents at site

Process Flow for obtaining Informed Consent Document from Illiterates

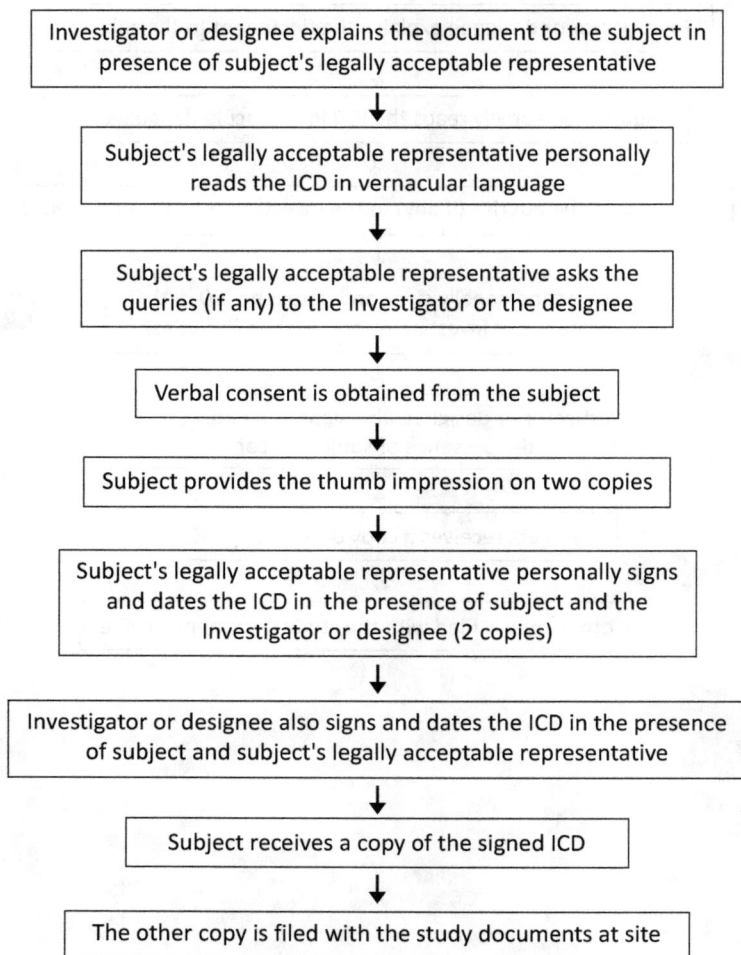

Investigator or designee explains the document to the subject in presence of subject's legally acceptable representative

↓

Subject's legally acceptable representative personally reads the ICD in vernacular language

↓

Subject's legally acceptable representative asks the queries (if any) to the Investigator or the designee

↓

Verbal consent is obtained from the subject

↓

Subject provides the thumb impression on two copies

↓

Subject's legally acceptable representative personally signs and dates the ICD in the presence of subject and the Investigator or designee (2 copies)

↓

Investigator or designee also signs and dates the ICD in the presence of subject and subject's legally acceptable representative

↓

Subject receives a copy of the signed ICD

↓

The other copy is filed with the study documents at site

Process Flow for obtaining Informed Consent Document when both Subject and Subject's Legally Acceptable Representative are Illiterate

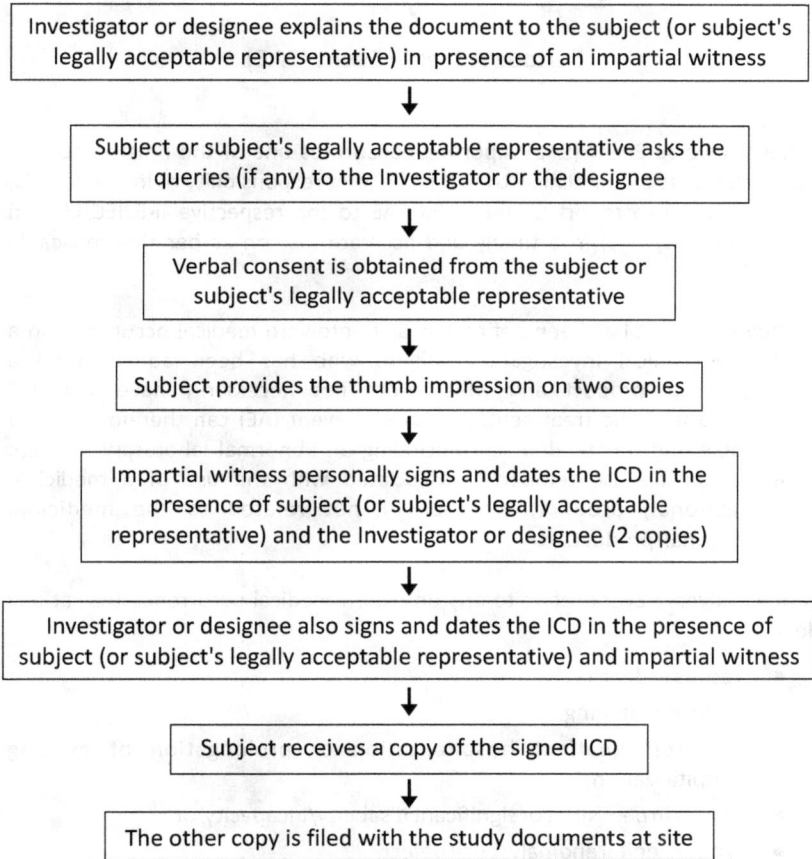

Investigator or designee explains the document to the subject (or subject's legally acceptable representative) in presence of an impartial witness

↓

Subject or subject's legally acceptable representative asks the queries (if any) to the Investigator or the designee

↓

Verbal consent is obtained from the subject or subject's legally acceptable representative

↓

Subject provides the thumb impression on two copies

↓

Impartial witness personally signs and dates the ICD in the presence of subject (or subject's legally acceptable representative) and the Investigator or designee (2 copies)

↓

Investigator or designee also signs and dates the ICD in the presence of subject (or subject's legally acceptable representative) and impartial witness

↓

Subject receives a copy of the signed ICD

↓

The other copy is filed with the study documents at site

9

Serious Adverse Event (SAE)

Serious Adverse Event (SAE) reporting constitutes one of the most important safety elements of any clinical trial. It is the joint responsibility of investigator(s) and sponsor(s) to report all the valid SAE to the respective IRB/IEC/EC and regulatory body (ies) in a timely and accurate fashion as per the applicable regulations.

An Adverse Event has been defined as any untoward medical occurrence in a patient or clinical investigation subject who has been administered a pharmaceutical product and which does not necessarily have a casual relationship with the treatment. An adverse event (AE) can therefore be any unfavorable and unintended sign (including an abnormal laboratory finding), symptom, or disease temporally associated with the use of a medicinal (investigational) product, whether or not related to the medicinal (investigational) product.

Serious Adverse Event refers to any untoward medical occurrence that at any dose:

- results in death,
- is life-threatening,
- requires inpatient hospitalization or prolongation of existing hospitalization,
- results in persistent or significant disability/incapacity, or
- is a congenital anomaly/birth defect,
- is considered serious by the investigator for a reason other than those listed.

In the event of an occurrence of a serious adverse reaction the patient shall be taken-off the study drug immediately. He/She shall be followed up for the adverse event even after the therapy discontinuation until the event or its sequel resolves or stabilize at a level acceptable to the investigator.

NOTE: The term "life-threatening" in the definition of "serious" refers to an event in which the patient is at risk of death at the time of the event, it does not refer to an event, which hypothetically might have caused death if it were more severe.

Medical and scientific judgment should be exercised in deciding whether expedited reporting is appropriate in other situations, such as important medical events that may not be immediately life-threatening or result in death or hospitalization but may jeopardize the patient or may require intervention to prevent one of the other outcomes listed in the definition above. These should also usually be considered serious.

Examples of such events are intensive treatment in an emergency room or at home for allergic bronchospasm; blood dyscrasias or convulsions that do not result in hospitalization; or development of drug dependency or drug abuse.

A distinction should be drawn between serious and severe experience. A severe experience is a major experience of its type. A severe experience need not necessarily be serious. For example, nausea, which persists for several hours, may be considered severe but not a serious adverse experience. On the other hand, a stroke, which results in, only a limited degree of disability may be considered a mild stroke but would be a serious adverse experience. The investigator is responsible for ensuring that there are procedures and expertise available to cope with medical emergencies during the study.

Before considering any clinical incident for submission to the FDA in an expedited or periodic safety report, applicants, manufacturers, and licensed manufacturers should have following four data elements to qualify it for a valid case:

1. an identifiable patient;
2. an identifiable reporter;
3. a suspect drug or biological product; and
4. an adverse event or fatal outcome

SAE Reporting Timelines (ICH-GCP)

From	To	Reporting Timelines
Investigator	Sponsor	Immediately
Investigator	Ethics Committee	As per the applicable regulatory requirements
Sponsor	Regulatory Authority	Fatal or life-threatening unexpected adverse drug reactions within 7 calendar days (initial report) and within 8 additional calender days (complete report)
		All other serious, unexcepted adverse drug reactions within 15 calender days.

ICH GCP guidelines specifies the SAE reporting timelines for various stakeholders and the same has been widely accepted by the regulatory authorities worldwide. In addition, there may be some country specific requirements that needs to be checked before initiating a clinical trial in that country.

SAE Reporting Process Flow - Investigator's Responsibilities

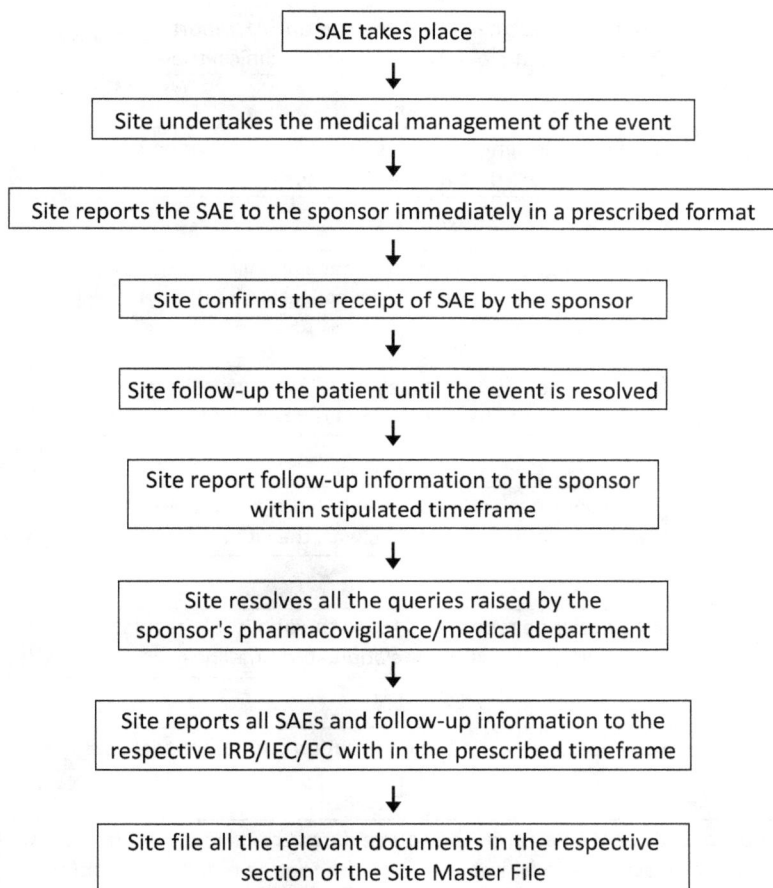

SAE takes place

↓

Site undertakes the medical management of the event

↓

Site reports the SAE to the sponsor immediately in a prescribed format

↓

Site confirms the receipt of SAE by the sponsor

↓

Site follow-up the patient until the event is resolved

↓

Site report follow-up information to the sponsor within stipulated timeframe

↓

Site resolves all the queries raised by the sponsor's pharmacovigilance/medical department

↓

Site reports all SAEs and follow-up information to the respective IRB/IEC/EC with in the prescribed timeframe

↓

Site file all the relevant documents in the respective section of the Site Master File

SAE Reporting Process Flow - Sponsor's Responsibilities

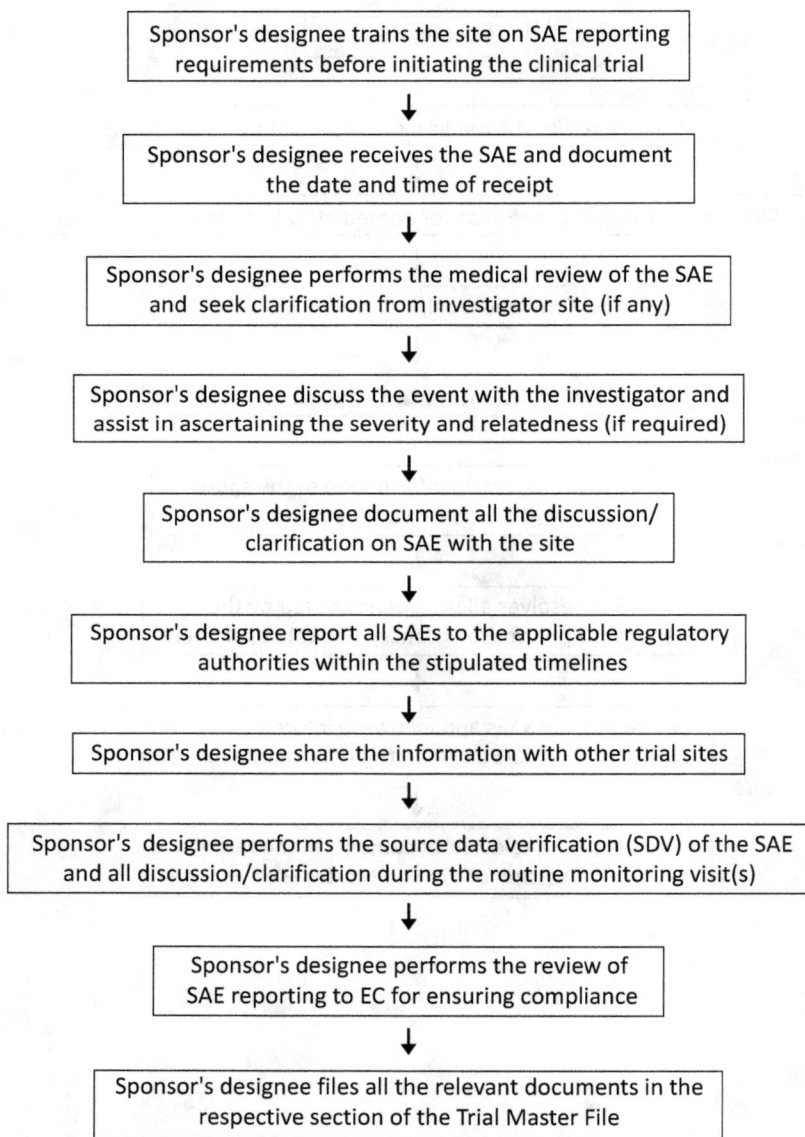

Sponsor's designee trains the site on SAE reporting requirements before initiating the clinical trial

↓

Sponsor's designee receives the SAE and document the date and time of receipt

↓

Sponsor's designee performs the medical review of the SAE and seek clarification from investigator site (if any)

↓

Sponsor's designee discuss the event with the investigator and assist in ascertaining the severity and relatedness (if required)

↓

Sponsor's designee document all the discussion/ clarification on SAE with the site

↓

Sponsor's designee report all SAEs to the applicable regulatory authorities within the stipulated timelines

↓

Sponsor's designee share the information with other trial sites

↓

Sponsor's designee performs the source data verification (SDV) of the SAE and all discussion/clarification during the routine monitoring visit(s)

↓

Sponsor's designee performs the review of SAE reporting to EC for ensuring compliance

↓

Sponsor's designee files all the relevant documents in the respective section of the Trial Master File

SAE REPORTING FORM (CIOMS-EMEA)

Suspect Adverse Reaction Report													

I. Reaction Information

I. Patient Initials (first, last)	I a. Country	2. Date of Birth			2. Age Years	3. Sex	4-6. Reaction onset			8-12 Check all Appropriate to adverse Reaction
		DD	MM	YY			DD	MM	YY	☐ Patient Died

7+13 Describe Reaction(s) (including relevanttests/lab data)	☐ Involved or Prolonged Inpatient Hospitalization
	☐ Involved persistence or significant Disability or incapacity
Narrative:*	☐ Life Threatening

II. Suspect Drug(s) Information

14. Suspect Drug(s) (include generic name)	20. Did Reaction Abate After Stopping Drug?
	☐Yes ☐No ☐NA

15. Daily Dose(s)	16. Route(s) of Administration	21. Did Reaction Reappear After Introduction?
17. Indication(s) for Use		
18. Therapy Dates (from/to)	19. Therapy Duration	☐Yes ☐No ☐NA

III. Concomitant Drugs and History

22. Concomitant Drug(s) and dates of administration (exclude those use to treat reaction)
23. Other Relevant history (*e.g.* diagnostics, allergics, pregnancy with last month of period, *etc.*)

IV. Manufacturer Information

24a. Name and Address of Manufacturer	
	24b. Mfr Control no.
24c. Date Received by Manufacturer	24d. Report Source ☐ Study ☐ Literature ☐ Health Professional
Date of this report	25a. Report type ☐ Initial ☐ Followup

SAE REPORTING FORM (US FDA-3500A)

U.S. Department of Health and Human Services
Food and Drug Administration

MEDWATCH

FORM FDA 3500A (6/10)

For use by user-facilities,
importers, distributors and manufacturerers
for MANDATORY reporting

Mfr Report#

UF/Importer Report#

FDA Use Only

A. PATIENT INFORMATION

1. Patient Identifier	2. Age at Time of Event : or _____ Date of Birth :	3. Sex	4. Weight
In confidence		☐ Female ☐ Male	_____ lbs or _____ kgs

B. ADVERSE EVENT OR PRODUCT PROBLEM

1. ☐ Adverse Event and/or ☐ Product Problem (e.g., defects/malfunctions)

2. Outcomes Attributed to Adverse Event (Check all that apply)

☐ Death _____ (mm/dd/yyyy)
☐ Life-threatening
☐ Hospitalization - initial or prolonged
☐ Required Intervention to Prevent Permanent Impairment/Damage (Devices)
☐ Disability or Permanent Damage
☐ Congenital Anomaly/Birth Defect
☐ Other Serious (Important Medical Events)

3. Date of Event (mm/dd/yyyy)

4. Date of This Report (mm/dd/yyyy)

5. Describe Event or Problem

6. Relevant Tests/Laboratory Data, Including Dates

7. Other Relevant History, Including Preexisting Medical Conditions (e.g., allergies, race, pregnancy, smoking and alcohol use, hepatic/renal dysfunction, etc.)

C. SUSPECT PRODUCT(S)

1. Name (Give labled strength & mfr/labeler)

#1
#2

2. Dose, Frequency & Route Used	3. Therapy Dates(If unknown, give duration) from/to (or best estimate)
#1	#1
#2	#2

4. Diagnosis for Use (Indication)	7. Event Abated After Use Stopped or Dose Reduced?
#1	#1 ☐ Yes ☐ No ☐ Doesn't Apply
#2	#2 ☐ Yes ☐ No ☐ Doesn't Apply

6. Lot #	7. Exp. Date	8. Event Reappeared After Reintroduction?
#1	#1	#1 ☐ Yes ☐ No ☐ Doesn't Apply
#2	#2	#2 ☐ Yes ☐ No ☐ Doesn't Apply

9. NDC # or Unique ID

10. Concomitant Medical Products and Therapy Dates (Exclude treatment of event)

D. SUSPECT MEDICAL DEVICE

1. Brand Name

2. Common Device Name

3. Manufacturer Name, City and State

4. Model #	Lot #	5. Operator of Device
Catalog #	Expiration Date (mm/dd./yy)	☐ Health Professional ☐ Lay User/Patient
Serial #	Other #	☐ Other:

6. If Implanted, Give Date (mm/dd/yyyy)	7. If Explanted, Give Date (mm/dd/yyyy)

8. Is this a Single-use Device that was Reprocessed and Reused on a Patient?
☐ Yes ☐ No

9. If Yes to Item No. 8, Enter Name and Address of Reprocessor

10. Device Available for Evaluation? (Do not send to FDA)
☐ Yes ☐ No ☐ Returned to Manufacturer on : _____ (mm/dd/yyyy)

11. Concomitant Medical Products and Therapy Dates (Exclude treatment of event)

E. INITIAL REPORTER

1. Name and Address	Phone #

2. Health Professional?	3. Occupation	4. Initial Reporter Also Sent Report to FDA
☐ Yes ☐ No		☐ Yes ☐ No ☐ Unk.

Submission of a report does not constitute and admission that medical Personnel, user facility, importer, distributor, manufacturer or product caused or contributed to the event.

MEDWATCH

FORM FDA 3500A (6/10) Continued

F. FOR USE BY USER FACILITY/IMPORTER (Devices Only)

1. Check One
☐ User facility ☐ Importer

2. UF/Importer Report Number

3. User Facility or Importer Name/Address

4. Contact Person

5. Phone Number

6. Date User Facility or Importer Became Aware of Event (mm/dd/yyyy)

7. Type of Report
☐ Initial
☐ Follow-up#_____

8. Date of This Report (mm/dd/yyyy)

9. Approximate Age of Device

10. Event Problem Codes (Refer to coding manual)
Patient Code ___ - ___ - ___
Device Code ___ - ___ - ___

11. Report Sent to FDA?
☐ Yes _____ (mm/dd/yyyy)
☐ No

12. Location Where Event Occurred
☐ Hospital
☐ Home
☐ Nursing Home
☐ Outpatient Treatment Facility
☐ Outpatient Diagnostic Facility
☐ Amulatory Surgical Facility
☐ Other: _____ (Specify)

13. Report Sent to Manufacturer?
☐ Yes _____ (mm/dd/yyyy)
☐ No

14. Manucacturer Name/Address

G. ALL MANUFACTURERS

1. Contact Office - Name/Address (and Manufacturing Site for Devices)

2. Phone Number

3. Report Source (Check all apply)
☐ Foreign
☐ Study
☐ Literature
☐ Consumer
☐ Health Professional
☐ User Facility
☐ Company Representative
☐ Distributor
☐ Other

4. Date Received by Manufacturer (mm/dd/yyyy)

5.
(A) NDA # _____
IND # _____
STN # _____
PMA/510(k) # _____
Combination Product ☐ Yes
Pre-1938 ☐ Yes
OTC Product ☐ Yes

6. If IND, Give Protocol #

7. Type of Report (Check all that apply)
☐ 5-day ☐ 30 day
☐ 7-day ☐ Periodic
☐ 10-day ☐ Initial
☐ 15-day ☐ Follow-up#_____

9. Manufacturer Report Number

8. Adverse Event Term(s)

H. DEVICE MANUCACTURERS ONLY

1. Type of Reportable Event
☐ Death
☐ Serious Injury
☐ Malfunction
☐ Other _____

2. If Follow-up, What Type?
☐ Correction
☐ Additional Information
☐ Response to FDA Request
☐ Device Evaluation

3. Device Evaluated by Manufacturer?
☐ Not Returned to Manufacturer
☐ Yes ☐ Evaluation Summary Attached
☐ No (Attach page to explain why not) or provide code : _____

4. Device Manufacture Date (mm/yyyy)

5. Labeled for Single Use?
☐ Yes ☐ No

6. Evaluation Codes (Refer to coding manual)
Method ___ - ___ - ___ - ___
Results ___ - ___ - ___ - ___
Conclusions ___ - ___ - ___

7. If Remedial Action Initiated, Check Type
☐ Recall   ☐ Notification
☐ Repair   ☐ Inspection
☐ Replace   ☐ Patient Monitoring
☐ Relabeling   ☐ Modification/Adjustment
☐ Other: _____

8. Usage of Device
☐ Initial Use of Device
☐ Reuse
☐ Unknown

9. If action reported to FDA under 21 USC 360I(f), list correction/removal reporting number:

10. ☐ Additional Manufacturer Narrative and/or **11.** ☐ Corrected Data

---

The public reporting burden for this collection of information has been estimated to average 66 minutes per response. including the time for reviewing instructions, searching existing data sources, gathering and maintaining the data needed, completing and reviewing the collection of information. Send comments regarding this burden estimated or any other aspect of this

Department of Health and Human Services
Food and Drug Administration
Office of Chief Information Officer
1350 Piccard Drive, Room 400
Rockville, MD 20850
Please DO NOT RETURN this form to this address.

MEDWATCH

FORM FDA 3500A (6/10) Continued

For use by user-facilities,
importers, distributors and manufacturerers
for MANDATORY reporting

B.5. Describe Event or Problem (Continued)

B.6. Relevant Tests/Laboratory Data, Including Dates (Continued)

B.7. Other Relevant History, Including Preexisting Medical Conditions (*e.g.*, allergies, race, pregnancy, smoking and alcohol use, hepatic/renal dysfunction, etc.) (Continued)

Concomitant Medical Products and Therapy Dates (Exclude treatment of event) (For continuation of C. 10 and/or D. 11; please distinguish) (Continued)

Other Remarks

10

Maintenance of Source Document

According to ICH-GCP, source document refers to original documents, data and records (*e.g.* hospital records, clinical and office charts, laboratory notes, memoranda, subject's diaries or evaluation check list, pharmacy dispensing records, recorded data from automated instruments, copies or transcriptions certified after verification as being accurate copies, micro fiches, photographic negatives, microfilm or magnetic media, X-rays, subject files and records kept at the pharmacy, at the laboratories and at medico-technical departments involved in the clinical trial).

It is the responsibility of investigator site to maintain the source document for each trial patient. Source document should be able to tell the complete story and one should be able to reconstruct the entire trial simply on the basis of information captured in the source document. All the information should be accurately recorded in the source document along with an audit trail of who did what and when it was done. It is a good practice to highlight a patient's participation in a clinical trial on the cover page of the source document.

The use of Case Report Forms (CRFs) as source document should be limited only to certain parameters like quality of life questionnaires, evaluation scales, patient demographics *etc.* and it should be mentioned in the study protocol.

A good source document should be able to address the following:

- ICD process,
- Pre-existing conditions and relevant history,
- Laboratory reports and results,
- Efficacy evaluations *e.g.* radiological investigations, blood glucose monitoring, patient's response *etc.,*
- Adverse events and corrective medications,
- Drug accountability,
- Progress notes,
- Patient's status (ongoing) *etc.*

1. ICD Process

Since voluntary consent is mandatory for any clinical trial, ICD process should always be documented. This includes a mention of:

- Whether the patient is literate or illiterate,
- Who was the legal representative in case of illiterate patient,
- Who was the impartial witness in case of illiterate patient with no legal representative or illiterate legal representative,
- Which translation was used,
- The queries/questions that the patient/legal representative had asked.

If a patient withdraws the consent during the course of the trial, it should be recorded in the source document along with the reason (if any).

2. Pre-existing Conditions and Relevant Medical History

All pre-existing conditions and the relevant present and past medical history including therapy undergone by the patient with duration should be included at the time of taking the initial notes. This includes a mention of:

- Start date of pre-existing conditions,
- Severity grade of pre-existing conditions,
- Corrective medications for pre-existing conditions,
- Stop date of significant historical diagnosis.

These should be followed up at every visit.

3. Laboratory Reports and Results

The laboratory results are the important safety parameters for assessing the side effects of the investigational product. All the laboratory reports and results should be maintained properly since this is a focus area during regulatory inspections.

- All lab reports should be placed in chronological order and should be duly signed by the reporter and the investigator/designee,
- All values that are out of reference range should be commented upon if they are clinically significant,
- Any dosing decision related to laboratory values should be taken only after the investigator/designee has reviewed, noted his comments and signed the lab reports,
- Use of whitener for obscuring the values should be avoided,
- Thermal printouts (from the automated machines) should be xeroxed and

enclosed along with the lab reports for providing an audit trail.

4. Efficacy Evaluations

While the safety is assessed using the laboratory results, efficacy is assessed with the help of the relevant diagnostic evaluation or from the patient's response when relevant diagnostic evaluation is not available. It includes radiological investigations for oncology trials; blood glucose monitoring for diabetes trials and patient's response for psychiatry trials *etc.*

Radiological investigations

- It should be on the same format, covering the same area across visits,
- All reports should be placed in chronological order and should be duly signed by the reporter and the investigator/designee,
- The films should be present in original and should not be physically altered *e.g.* bent/ folded/ cut.

Blood glucose monitoring

- All reports should be placed in chronological order and should be duly signed by the reporter and the investigator/designee,
- Patient's response should be verifiable from the diaries/cards/ glucometers.

Patient's response

- It should be collected in diaries/cards/ questionnaires,
- Appropriate translation of the diaries/cards/questionnaires should be used,
- Diaries/cards/questionnaires should be present in original at trial site.

5. Adverse Events and Corrective Medications

- All Adverse events occurring during the course of study should be recorded with the respective start and stop dates,
- Each adverse event should be recorded with the grade of severity,
- Adverse events should be followed-up every time the patient's visit takes place,
- Patient should be evaluated for new adverse event(s) at every visit,
- Medication once started by patient should be followed-up at every visit until it is stopped,
- Dose/frequency of each medication should be documented,

- Start and stop date of each medication should be clearly stated in the patient file,
- Any change in the dosage/frequency of the medication should be documented in the patient's file.

6. Drug Accountability

- 100 % drug accountability is must at all levels,
- Number of units of each batch number of the drug(s) dispensed to the patient(s) at every visit should be documented,
- Number of units of each batch number of the drug(s) returned during each visit (if applicable) should be documented,
- Any discrepancy (breakage/loss/damage) should be properly documented.

7. Progress Notes

- Patient's medical/progress notes should include details about the patient's medical condition and well-being across visits,
- For unscheduled/telephonic visits progress notes should be incorporated in the patient file.

8. Patient's Status (ongoing)

- Patient's status/condition should be recorded on an ongoing basis,
- If the patient is referred to another department/hospital; all the relevant details should be recorded in the source document,
- If the patient becomes lost to follow-up, all communications/attempts to contact the patient should be mentioned in the patient file.

All Source Documents should be archived for appropriate duration of time. If the institutional archival time is less than the trial requirements a special note should be mentioned on individual source document and the medical record section should be sensitized about it.

As trial patient requires a frequent follow-up, most of the investigators retain the source document of trial patients with them and a note in this regard is generally kept at the medical record section.

If electronic media is used for creating and/or storing source data proper care should be taken for ensuring the security, validation and back up control mechanism.

Tips on Maintaining the Source Document

1. Ensure that
☞ the protocol number is mentioned on the patient file to highlight the clinical trial participation

☞ the protocol number is present on the prescription form

☞ all entries in worksheets or patient files has date and initials of person making the entry

> **Proper access control should exist for the source document, which should be able to address "who did what" and "when it was done"**

2. Document
☞ the date patient gave consent, with the protocol number

☞ the date the initial discussions took place if different from the consent date

☞ the consent process (whether the patient is literate or illiterate, who were the witness and which translation was used)

☞ the date the patient withdrew consent with reason (if any)

> **Voluntary consent is essential for protecting the rights, safety and well being of trial subject(s)**

3. Make entries of
☞ the number of units of each batch number of the investigational product dispensed to the patient(s) at scheduled visits

☞ the number of units of each batch number of the investigational product returned during each scheduled visit (if applicable)

☞ any discrepancy (breakage/ loss/ damage)

> **Documentation of all the transaction of the study drug would lead to 100% drug accountability**

4. Always makes sure that
☞ all the records of a patient are filed together in one file

☞ if the patient is referred to another department/hospital, all the relevant records are included in the source document

☞ all diagnostic reports are duly signed and filed together in a chronological order

- ☞ all patient records/notes are together and in continuity
- ☞ start and stop date for all adverse event(s) and corrective medication(s) are clearly stated in the patient file

Incomplete and inappropriate source document(s) can lead to significant audit issues

5. Find out

- ☞ where the source document(s) are kept once the study is over or after the patient's death
- ☞ how the source document(s) are kept (*e.g.* environmental protection from fire, flood, termite *etc.*)

All Source Documents are required to be archived for a specified period of time (10-15 years) after the completion of trial for the purpose of audit/inspection.

Source Document Don'ts

- ➢ Use of Xerox copy of CRF as source document
- ➢ Creation of trial specific source document
- ➢ Missing data/entries in the source document
- ➢ Changes to data questionable (signatures of the person making the changes missing)
- ➢ Disorganized records and data for a patient kept in separate files
- ➢ Inappropriate filing of patient notes/reports
- ➢ Messy documentation
- ➢ Lack of access control
- ➢ Source document discarded after the trial is over

11

IND, NDA, ANDA and AADA

Investigational New Drug (IND) Application

After completing preclinical testing, a company/organization files an IND with FDA to begin the test of drug in Human. INDA (Investigational New Drug Application) is the means through which sponsor (usually the manufacturer or potential marketer) obtain a legal status to call its new investigational molecule as new drug. The IND is not an application for marketing approval. During the IND review process, the medical reviewer evaluates the clinical trial protocol to determine:

- if the participants will be protected from unnecessary risks; and
- if the study design will provide data relevant to the safety and effectiveness of the drug.

The IND becomes effective if FDA does not disapprove it within 30 days. The IND shows results of previous experiments, how, where and by whom the new studies will be conducted; the chemical structure of the compound; mechanism of action of the compound; any toxic effects found in the animal studies; and how the compound is manufactured. In addition, the IND must be reviewed and approved by the Institutional Review Board where the studies will be conducted, and progress reports on clinical trials must be submitted at least annually to FDA.

Main components of an IND are:

- description of the drug substance
- chemistry, manufacturing and control information
- all known pre-clinical information
- any previous human study reports
- investigator's brochure
- clinical development plan
- protocol and investigator list

Each time a new study protocol or new study site is initiated or added to an ongoing protocol, the IND must be amended. Protocol amendments also require an amendment to the IND. The FDA has 30 days to respond to the sponsor's IND.

Categories of IND

Commercial and Non Commercial (Research)

"Commercial INDs" are applications that are submitted primarily by companies whose ultimate goal is to obtain marketing approval for a new product. However, there is another class of filings broadly known as **"Non-commercial" INDs**. The vast majority of INDs are, in fact, filed for non-commercial research. These types of INDs include "Investigator INDs," "Emergency Use INDs," and "Treatment INDs."

- **Investigator IND** is submitted by a physician who both initiates and conducts an investigation, and under whose immediate direction the investigational drug is administered or dispensed. A physician might submit a research IND to propose studying an unapproved drug, or an approved product for a new indication or in a new patient population. In this case, the physician is both the sponsor and investigator. Usually the investigator will cross-reference the original sponsor companies IND for the pre clinical and clinical information.

- **Emergency Use IND:** The FDA can authorize immediate dispensing of a non-approved drug in a life-threatening situation when no standard acceptable therapy is available and there is not enough time to obtain IRB approval. This may also be referred to as "compassionate use" IND.

- **Treatment IND:** Non-approved drugs showing promise in clinical testing for treatment of serious or life-threatening conditions are made available while the final clinical work and the FDA review is still ongoing. FDA will permit an investigational drug to be used under a treatment IND if there is preliminary evidence of drug efficacy and the drug is intended to treat a serious or life-threatening disease, or if there is no comparable alternative drug or therapy available to treat that stage of the disease in the intended patient population. An immediately life-threatening disease means a stage of a disease in which there is a reasonable likelihood that death will occur within a matter of months or in which premature death is likely without early treatment. For *e.g.*, advanced cases of AIDS, herpes simplex encephalitis, and subarachnoid hemorrhage are all considered to be immediately life-threatening diseases. Treatment INDs are made available to patients before general marketing begins, typically during Phase 3 studies. Treatment INDs also allow FDA to obtain additional data on the drug's safety.

The IND application (FDA 1571) must contain information on three broad areas:

- **Animal Pharmacology and Toxicology Studies**: Preclinical data to permit an assessment as to whether the product is reasonably safe for initial testing in humans.

- **Manufacturing Information**: Information pertaining to the composition, manufacturer, stability, and controls used for manufacturing the drug substance and the drug product. This information is assessed to ensure that the company can adequately produce and supply consistent batches of the drug.
- **Clinical Protocols and Investigator Information**: Detailed protocols for proposed clinical studies to assess whether the initial-phase trials will expose subjects to unnecessary risks. Also, information on the qualifications of clinical investigators professionals (generally physicians) who oversee the administration of the experimental compound to assess whether they are qualified to fulfill their clinical trial duties. Finally, commitments to obtain informed consent from the research subjects, to obtain review of the study by an institutional review board (IRB), and to adhere to the investigational new drug regulations.

New Drug Application (NDA)

NDA is an application submitted to the FDA for permission to market a new drug product. To obtain this permission, a drug manufacturer/sponsor submits in the NDA, non-clinical (animal) and clinical (human) test data and analyses, drug information, and descriptions of manufacturing procedures.

Fundamentals of NDA Submissions

Although the quantity of information and data submitted in NDAs can vary significantly, the components of NDAs are more uniform. The components of any NDA are, in part, a function of the nature of the subject drug and the information available to the applicant at the time of submission. NDAs can consist of as many as 15 different sections:

- index,
- summary,
- chemistry, manufacturing, and control,
- samples, methods validation package, and labeling,
- non-clinical pharmacology and toxicology,
- human pharmacokinetics and bioavailability,
- microbiology (for anti-microbial drugs only),
- clinical data,
- safety update report (typically submitted 120 days after the NDA's submission),
- statistical,
- case report tabulations,
- case report forms,

- patent information,
- patent certification and
- other information.

NDA Content and Format Requirements

The NDA must provide all relevant data and information that a sponsor has collected during the product's research and development though the exact requirements depends on the nature of a specific drug. The FDA has numerous guidelines that relate to NDA content and format issues which can be found on its website.

NDA Classifications

New Drug Applications are being classified by FDA with a code that reflects both the type of drug being submitted and its intended uses. The numbers 1 through 7 are used to describe the type of drug:

1. new molecular entity,
2. new salt of previously approved drug (not a new molecular entity),
3. new formulation of previously approved drug (not a new salt or a new molecular entity),
4. new combination of two or more drugs,
5. already marketed drug product - duplication (*i.e.*, new manufacturer),
6. new indication (claim) for already marketed drug (includes switch in marketing status from prescription to OTC),
7. already marketed drug product - not previously approved NDA.

The following letter codes describe the review priority of the drug:

S- Standard review for drugs similar to currently available drugs

P- Priority review for drugs that represent significant advances over existing treatments

After a New Drug Application (NDA) is received by the agency, it undergoes a technical screening generally referred to as a completeness review. This evaluation ensures that sufficient data and information have been submitted in each area to justify "filing" the application that is, justifying initiating FDA formal review of the NDA.

At the conclusion of NDA review by the FDA, there are three possible action letters that can be sent to the sponsor:

- **Not Approvable letter** lists the deficiencies in the application and explains why the application cannot be approved.
- **Approvable letter** signals that, ultimately, the drug can be approved. Lists minor deficiencies that can be corrected, often involves labeling changes, and possibly requests commitment to do post-approval studies.
- **Approval letter** states that the drug is approved. May follow an approvable letter, but can also be issued directly.

If the action taken is either an approvable or a not approvable action (as opposed to an approval action), FDA provides applicants with an opportunity to meet with agency officials and discuss the deficiencies. The purpose of the meeting is to discuss what further steps are necessary before the application can be approved.

The goals of the NDA are to provide enough information to permit FDA reviewer to reach the following key decisions:

☑ Whether the drug is safe and effective in its proposed use(s), and whether the benefits of the drug outweigh the risks.

☑ Whether the drug's proposed labeling (package insert) is appropriate, and what it should contain.

☑ Whether the methods used in manufacturing the drug and the controls used to maintain the drug's quality are adequate to preserve the drug's identity, strength, quality, and purity.

Abbreviated New Drug Application (ANDA) and Abbreviated Antibiotic Drug Application (AADA)

An Abbreviated New Drug Application (ANDA) and Abbreviated Antibiotic Drug Application (AADA) is submitted to FDA's Center for Drug Evaluation and Research, Office of Generic Drugs to obtain the approval to market a generic drug product. It contains data which when approved makes an applicant eligible to manufacture and market the generic drug product as a safe, effective and low cost alternative.

Generic drug applications are termed "abbreviated" because they are generally not required to include preclinical (animal) and clinical (human) data to establish safety and effectiveness. Instead, generic applicants must scientifically demonstrate that their product is bioequivalent (*i.e.*, performs in the same manner as the innovator drug).

Use of bioequivalence studies as the basis for the approval of generic drug products was established by the "Drug Price Competition and Patent Term Restoration Act of 1984" also known as the Waxman-Hatch Act. This Act expedites the availability of less costly generic drugs by permitting FDA to approve applications to market generic versions of the innovator drugs without conducting costly and duplicative clinical trials. A generic drug product is one that is comparable to an innovator drug product in dosage form, strength, route of administration, quality, performance characteristics and intended use. All approved products, both innovator and generic, are listed in FDA's Approved Drug Products with Therapeutic Equivalence Evaluations (Orange Book).

Generic drug application (FDA 356h) reviewers focus on bioequivalence data, chemistry and microbiology data, requests for plant inspection, and drug labeling information. ANDA must contain sufficient information to allow a review to be conducted in an efficient and timely manner. If one or more essential components is missing, a Refuse to File letter is issued to the applicant. The letter identifies the missing component(s) and informs the applicant that the application will not be filed until it is complete.

Bioequivalence Review

FDA requires an ANDA applicant to provide information to establish bioequivalency. Such information may include:

- formulation comparison for products whose bioavailability is self evident, for *e.g.*, oral solutions, injectables, or ophthalmic solutions where the formulations are identical;
- comparative dissolution testing where there is a known correlation between in vitro and in vivo effects;
- in vivo bioequivalence testing comparing the rate and extent of absorption of the generic to the reference product;
- and for non-classically absorbed products, a head-to-head evaluation of comparative effectiveness based upon clinical endpoints.

If the bioequivalence review determines that there are deficiencies in the bioequivalence portion of the application, then a bioequivalence deficiency letter is issued to the applicant. The deficiency letter will detail the deficiencies and request information and data to resolve the deficiencies. If the review determines the bioequivalence portion of the application is acceptable, a letter indicating that there are no further questions at that time will be issued.

ANDA/AADA Approval

After the review of all components of an ANDA, an approval or tentative letter may be issued to the applicant detailing the conditions of the approval and providing them with the ability to market the generic drug product. If the approval occurs prior to the expiration of any patents or exclusivities accorded to the reference listed drug product, a tentative approval letter is issued to the applicant which details the tentative approval of the generic drug product until the patent/exclusivity condition has expired. A tentative approval does not allow the applicant to market the generic drug product.

Appendix I - List and Location of Essential Trial Documents Before the Clinical Phase of the Trial Commences

Sl. No.	Title of the Document	Located in files of			
		Investigator	Sponsor	CRO	IRB
1.	Investigator's brochure	✓	✓	✓	✓
2.	Signed protocol and amendments, if any, and sample case report form (CRF)	✓	✓	✓	✓
3.	Information given to trial subject - Informed consent form (including all applicable translations) - Any other written information - Advertisement for subject recruitment (if used)	✓	✓	✓	✓
4.	Financial aspects of the trial	✓	✓	✓	✓
5.	Insurance statement	✓	✓	✓	✓
6.	Dated, documented approval/ favorable opinion of institutional review board (IRB) of the following: - Protocol and any amendments - CRF (if applicable) - Informed consent form(s) - Any other written information to be provided to the subject(s) - Advertisement for subject recruitment (if used) - Subject compensation (if any)	✓	✓	✓	✓
7.	Institutional review board/Independent ethics committee composition	✓	✓	✓	✓

Sl. No.	Title of the Document	Located in files of			
		Investigator	Sponsor	CRO	IRB
8.	Regulatory authority (ies) authorization/approval/ notification of protocol (where required)	✓	✓	✓	✓
9.	Curriculum vitae and/or other relevant documents evidencing qualifications of investigator(s) and Co-investigator(s)/ Sub-Investigator(s)	✓	✓	✓	✓
10.	Normal value(s)/range(s) for medical/laboratory/technical procedure(s) and/or test(s) included in the protocol	✓	✓	✓	X
11.	Sample of label(s) attached to investigational product container(s)	X	✓	✓	X
12.	Instructions for handling of investigational product(s) and trial-related materials (if not included in protocol or Investigator's Brochure)	✓	✓	✓	X
13.	Shipping records for investigational product(s) and trial-related materials	✓	✓	✓	X
14.	Certificate(s) of analysis of investigational product(s) shipped	X	✓	✓	X
15.	Master randomization list	X	✓	✓	X
16.	Pre-trial monitoring report	X	✓	✓	X
17.	Trial initiation monitoring report	✓	✓	✓	X
18.	Decoding procedures for blinded trials	✓	✓	✓	X

Sl. No.	Title of the Document	Located in files of			
		Investigator	Sponsor	CRO	IRB
19.	Signed Agreement between involved parties - Investigator/institution and Sponsor - Investigator/institution and CRO - Sponsor and CRO - Investigator/institution and Authority(ies) [where required]	✓ ✓ X ✓	✓ ✓ ✓ ✓	✓ ✓ ✓ ✓	✓ ✓ X X
20.	Medical/Laboratory/Technical procedures/ Tests - Certification or - Accreditation or - Established quality control and/or external quality assessment or other validation (where required)	✓	✓	✓	X

Appendix II - List and Location of Essential Trial Documents During the Clinical Conduct of a Trial

Sl. No.	Title of the Document	Located in files of			
		Investigator	Sponsor	CRO	IRB
1.	Investigator's brochure updates	✓	✓	✓	✓
2.	Any revision to: - Protocol/protocol amendment(s) and CRF - Informed consent form - Any other written information provided to subjects - Advertisement for subject - Recruitment(if used)	✓	✓	✓	✓
3.	Dated, documented approval/ favorable opinion of institutional review board (IRB) of the following: - Protocol amendment(s) - Revision(s) of: - informed consent form - any other written information provided to subject - advertisement for subject recruitment(if used) - any other documents given approval/ favorable opinion continuing review of trial (where required)	✓	✓	✓	✓
4.	Regulatory authority(ies) authorizations/approvals/ notifications where required for: - Protocol amendment(s) and other documents	✓	✓	✓	✓
5.	Curriculum vitae for new Investigator(s) and/or Sub-investigator(s)	✓	✓	✓	✓

Sl. No.	Title of the Document	Located in files of			
		Investigator	Sponsor	CRO	IRB
6.	Updates to normal value(s)/ range(s) for medical/laboratory/ technical procedure(s)/test(s) included in the protocol	✓	✓	✓	X
7.	Updates of medical/laboratory/ technical procedures/tests - Certification or - Accreditation or - Established quality control and/or external quality assessment or other validation (where required)	✓	✓	✓	X
8.	Documentation of investigational product(s) and trial-related material shipment	✓	✓	✓	X
9.	Certificate(s) of analysis for new batches of investigational product(s)	X	✓	✓	X
10.	Monitoring visit report(s)	X	✓	✓	X
11.	Relevant communications other than site visits - Letters - Meeting notes - Notes of telephone calls	✓	✓	✓	X
12.	Signed informed consent forms	✓	X	X	X
13.	Source document(s)	✓	X	X	X
14.	Signed, dated and completed case report forms (CRF)	✓	✓	✓	X
15.	Documentation of CRF corrections	✓	✓	✓	X
16.	Notification from investigator of serious adverse events and related reports	✓	✓	✓	✓

Sl. No.	Title of the Document	Located in files of			
		Investigator	Sponsor	CRO	IRB
17.	Notification by sponsor and/or investigator, where applicable, to regulatory authority(ies) and IEC(s) of unexpected serious adverse drug reactions and of other safety information	✓	✓	✓	✓
18.	Notification by sponsor to investigators of safety information	✓	✓	✓	✓
19.	Interim or annual reports to IEC and authority(ies)	✓	✓	✓	✓
20.	Subject screening log	✓	✓	✓	X
21.	Subject identification code list	✓	X	X	X
22.	Subject enrolment log	✓	X	X	X
23.	Investigational product(s) accountability at the site	✓	✓	✓	X
24.	Signature sheet	✓	✓	✓	X
25.	Record of retained body fluids/ tissue samples (if any)	✓	✓	✓	X

**Appendix III - List and Location of Essential Trial Documents
After Completion or Termination of the Trial**

Sl. No.	Title of the Document	Located in files of			
		Investigator	Sponsor	CRO	IRB
1.	Investigational product(s) accountability at site	✓	✓	✓	X
2.	Documentation of investigational product destruction	✓ (if destroyed at site)	✓	✓	X
3.	Completed subject identification code list	✓	X	X	X
4.	Audit certificate (if available)	X	✓	✓	X
5.	Final trial close-out monitoring report	X	✓	✓	X
6.	Treatment allocation and decoding documentation	X	✓	✓	X
7.	Final report by investigator to IRB where required, and where applicable, to the regulatory authority(ies)	✓	X	X	✓
8.	Clinical study report	✓	✓	✓	X

References:

1. Drews J. Drug Discovery: a historical perspective. Science 2000; 287: 1960-64.

2. Julka P.K. 2011. Developing A World Class Clinical Trial Site. New Delhi: CR Books Pvt. Ltd. 163p.

3. Wax PM. 1995. Elixirs, diluents, and the passage of the 1938 Federal Food, Drug and Cosmetic Act. Annals of Internal Medicine 122: 456-61.

4. Diggle GE. 2001. Thalidomide: 40 years on. International Journal of Pharmaceutical Medicine 55: 627-31.

5. World Medical Association Declaration of Helsinki, Ethical Principles for Medical Research Involving Human Subjects, Adopted by the 18th WMA General Assembly Helsinki, Finland, June 1964 and its subsequent amendments.
Available from: http://www.wma.net/e/policy/b3.htm

6. http://www.ich.org [homepage on the Internet]: E6 (R1): Switzerland: Good Clinical Practice: Consolidated Guidelines.
Available from http://www.ich.org/LOB/media/MEDIA482.pdf

7. U.S. Food and Drug Administration [homepage on the Internet].
Available from www.fda.gov